C. J. Heath and E. G. Jones

The Anatomical Organization
of the Suprasylvian Gyrus
of the Cat

With 32 Figures

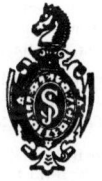

Springer-Verlag Berlin Heidelberg GmbH 1971

Dr. C. J. Heath* and Dr. E. G. Jones
Department of Anatomy
University of Otago Medical School
P.O. Box 913, Dunedin
New Zealand

* Present Address: University Laboratory of Physiology
Oxford, England

ISBN 978-3-540-05596-9   ISBN 978-3-642-48154-3 (eBook)
DOI 10.1007/978-3-642-48154-3

Contents

Abbreviations

A	anterior nuclei	*P*	posterior nucleus (Rioch, 1929)
Am	amygdala	*peV*	peristriate belt
As	anterior suprasylvian sulcus		(Sanides and Hoffmann, 1969)
AI	first auditory area	*Pl*	pulvinar
AII	second auditory area	*pL*	paralimbic region
AIII	third auditory area		(Sanides and Hoffmann, 1969)
B	brachium of inferior colliculus	*PLs*	postlateral sulcus
C	cingulate area	*Poi*	intermediate division of posterior
CL	central lateral nucleus		group
CM	centre médian nucleus	*Pol*	lateral division of posterior group
d	dorsal division of medial	*Pom*	medial division of posterior group
	geniculate body	*Ps*	posterior suprasylvian sulcus
Ep	posterior ectosylvian auditory area	*Pt*	parietal integration belt
GLd	dorsal lateral geniculate nucleus		(Sanides and Hoffmann, 1969)
GLv	ventral lateral geniculate nucleus	*R*	reticular nucleus
Ins	insular area	*Rs*	retrosplenial area
It	suprasylvian integration belt	*SF*	suprasylvian fringe
	(Sanides and Hoffmann, 1969)	*SG*	suprageniculate nucleus
Kv	visual koniocortex	*Ss*	suprasylvian sulcus belt
	(Sanides and Hoffmann, 1969)		(Sanides and Hoffmann, 1969)
L	n. limitans	*SI*	first somatic sensory area
LD	n. lateralis dorsalis	*SII*	second somatic sensory area
LM	medial lemniscus	*T*	taste areas
LP	n. lateralis posterior	*Te*	temporal auditory area
LS	lateral suprasylvian area	*TO*	optic tract
mc	magnocellular division of medial	*v*	ventral division of medial
	geniculate body		geniculate body
MD	medio-dorsal nucleus	*VA*	ventroanterior nucleus
mi	medial interlaminar nucleus of	*VL*	ventrolateral nucleus
	dorsal lateral geniculate nucleus	*VM*	ventromedial nucleus
Ms	middle suprasylvian sulcus	*VP*	ventroposterior nucleus
Not	nucleus of optic tract		

I. Introduction[1]

In recent years, the suprasylvian gyrus of the cat has attracted the attention of many neurophysiologists and experimental psychologists and the variety of their interests is reflected in the number of morphological and functional subdivisions which have been made of it. Some of these subdivisions are shown in Fig. 1. Workers concerned with the visual system have made studies of the third visual area (area 19) on the medial aspect of the gyrus, and of the lateral suprasylvian area on the lateral aspect, both of which contain representations of the retina (Clare and Bishop, 1954; Hubel and Wiesel, 1965, 1969; Wright, 1969). However, the full extent of these areas and particularly of the latter, is still not known. Other workers have investigated the extent of the gyrus activated by somatic sensory (Darian-Smith, Isbister, Mok and Yokota, 1966) or auditory (Woolsey, 1961) stimuli. A third field of increasing interest is the study of the "polysensory areas" of the cortex, two of which are situated in the middle suprasylvian gyrus. In these areas, in animals anaesthetized with chloralose, convergence upon single neurons of auditory, somatic and visual impulses has been demonstrated (see eg. Thompson, Johnson and Hoopes, 1963; Dubner and Rutledge, 1964, 1965; Dubner, 1966; Bignall, 1967) and it has been proposed that these areas play an important part in the central processing of sensory information (Buser and Bignall, 1967; Thompson, 1967). Although it has been shown that both subcortical and cortico-cortical mechanisms may determine the response properties of neurons in the polysensory areas (Dubner and Rutledge, 1965; Dubner and Brown, 1968; Bignall, 1967; Rutledge and Shellenberger, 1968) there is, as yet, no conclusive evidence of the pathways involved. Moreover, the polysensory areas have not been correlated with any known architectonic fields in the cat. It may be significant, however, that these areas are more or less coextensive with the regions in which occur: maximum barbiturate spindling, recruiting responses and responses to electrical stimulation of the midbrain reticular formation (Thompson, 1967).

The suprasylvian gyrus, thus, invites experimental anatomical study and the present investigation has a bearing on many of the spheres of interest mentioned above. However, a second aspect of the study may be of more general interest. With the exception of a very small frontal area, all of the association cortex possessed by the cat is situated in the middle and posterior suprasylvian gyri. Even here, the amount of cortex which may be considered "association cortex" in the usual sense, may be further restricted: the rostral part of the middle suprasylvian gyrus appears to be primarily related to the somatic sensory system and has even been called a "third somatic sensory area" (Darian-Smith, Isbister, Mok and Yokota, 1966); the medial and lateral surfaces of the gyrus contain the two visual areas, area 19 and the lateral suprasylvian area. The remaining "uncommitted cortex" is consequently very small. Yet the observations made on the brains of small mammals by earlier workers such as Brodmann (1909) and his followers suggest that approximately the same number of architectonic fields as are found in higher mammals should be situated here. It has sometimes been

---

1 Dedicated to Professor W. E. Adams on the occasion of his 63rd birthday.

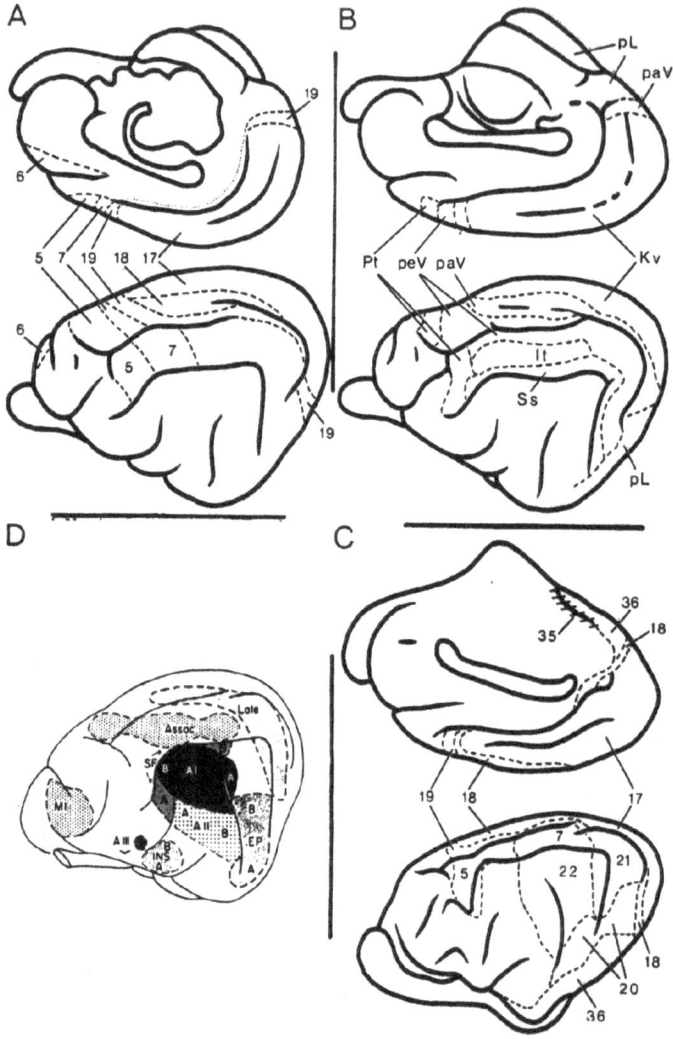

Fig. 1 A–D. Drawings of the cytoarchitectonic fields of the suprasylvian and adjacent regions of the cortex of the cat as delimited (A) by Hassler and Muhs-Clement (1964) and Otsuka and Hassler (1962); B by Sanides and Hoffmann (1969); C by Gurewitsch and Chatschaturian (1928). In A and C the architectonic fields are numbered following Brodmann (1909) while in B each is named (see text). D The evoked potential map of Woolsey (1961) showing the fields in which auditory responses may be evoked and the motor cortex (*MI*). The letters A and B in the auditory fields indicate the representations of the apical and basal portions of the cochlea

disclaimed that the architectonic subdivisions made by Brodmann and his school have much significance (Lashley and Clark, 1946; Bailey and Bonin, 1951). However, evidence is accruing to show that at least in the primary sensory areas of the cortex, architectonic subdivisions may be correlated with the response properties of their constituent neurons (Powell and Mountcastle, 1959; Hubel and Wiesel, 1965). Moreover, these and certain other architectonic fields have specific patterns of nervous connexions: both in being dependencies of specific thalamic nuclei (Rose and Woolsey, 1948a, b, 1949a, b; Le Gros Clark and Powell, 1952; Roberts and Akert, 1963) and in having different cortico-cortical relationships (Jones and Powell, 1968a, 1969a; Diamond, Jones and Powell, 1968a, 1969). The latter have been particularly studied in the monkey (Jones and Powell, 1970a) where the architectonic fields, in being larger, are more amenable to experimental analysis. In the monkey, it has been shown that from the point of view of cortico-cortical connexions, the significance of the architectonic fields of the parieto-temporal region could lie in their being successive steps in a sequence of cortical processing of sensory information emanating from the primary sensory areas. With this work on the monkey as a basis, it has been possible, within limits, to make a comparable analysis of the smaller suprasylvian association cortex of the cat and to draw certain parallels between the two species.

II. Material and Methods

This study is based upon experiments carried out in 56 adult cats. In 25, small unilateral lesions were made in known functional or architectonic fields of the cerebral cortex by removing a small portion of the pia mater, thus devascularizing the underlying cortex. Other, larger lesions were made in 5 cats with a suction aspirator and were regionally located only. In 16 cats, electrolytic lesions were made stereotaxically in the thalamus, using an electrode introduced horizontally from behind and entering the thalamus through the superior colliculus or the midbrain in order to avoid damage to the overlying cerebral cortex. In some cases, to avoid the corpus callosum, tentorium cerebelli or visual cortex, the electrode was given a slight upwards and/or lateral inclination. In 10 of this latter group of cats, the thalamic lesions were bilateral since the thalamo-cortical pathways involved are unilateral (Heath and Jones, 1971).

The animals were killed after 3 to 6 days by perfusion with formalin and the brains were sectioned at 25 μ on a freezing microtome. Alternate, one in ten or one in twenty series of sections were stained by the methods of Nauta and Gygax (1954) and of Fink and Heimer (1967) and over the extent of the thalamus and certain parts of the cortex further series were stained with thionin. The position of the lesions and the distribution of axonal degeneration in the cortex and thalamus were recorded on projection drawings of relevant sections and, in the case of the cortex, reconstructed on tracings of photographs of the individual brains. Sections from a number of normal brains stained with thionin were available for comparison. For convenience, all figures are presented as though the lesion were on the left side of the brain.

III. Results
General Considerations

Throughout these results, we shall be concerned to demonstrate three main aspects of the organization of the suprasylvian gyrus: (i) the extent of individual cortical areas delimited on the basis of their connexions; (ii) the relationships of these areas to one another and, particularly, to the primary sensory areas; (iii) the extent to which these areas may be correlated with known functional and architectonic subdivisions of the gyrus. In delimiting the boundaries of an area

we shall rely quite heavily on its intrinsic and its afferent cortico-cortical connexions as demonstrated by the axonal degeneration method. It has been shown
repeatedly that these connexions generally respect the boundaries of individual
cortical fields (Jones and Powell, 1968a; 1969a; Diamond, Jones and Powell,
1968a). In other words, if a lesion is localized within a given field, the ensuing
terminal degeneration in that field is confined to it, stopping abruptly at its
boundaries. Similarly, the terminal degeneration in one field following a lesion
of an adjoining or a more distant field, is confined within the boundaries of the
first field. The same is generally true of the cortical degeneration ensuing from a
lesion restricted to an individual thalamic nucleus, as will be demonstrated in the
first group of experiments to be described. However, because the suprasylvian
gyrus is related to a heterogeneous complex of thalamic nuclei, parts of which are
not readily subdivided on morphological criteria, and, more importantly, because
it has not been possible to devise a stereotaxic approach which would not simul-
taneously damage several parts of this complex, the distribution of degenerating
thalamo-cortical fibres has been useful mainly in confirming the boundaries of
fields delimited by other connexions. The results will be presented from the point
of view of the pathways whereby different types of sensory information may enter
the gyrus and the areas in which these different sensory inputs may converge.

Lack of Projections from the Thalamic Sensory Nuclei

The total extent of the neocortex which receives fibres from the nuclei of the
thalamus directly connected to the ascending somatic sensory, visual and auditory
pathways has been defined by experiments involving stereotaxic lesions of the
appropriate nuclei. As most of these experiments have been described in detail
in previous publications, they will be referred to only briefly (Fig. 2).

The Ventroposterior Nucleus. The cortical projection of the somatic sensory
relay nucleus, the ventroposterior, is confined to the first (SI) and second (SII)
somatic sensory areas, with extension into the taste areas lying below them in the
lateral bank of the presylvian sulcus (Burton and Earls, 1969; Jones and Powell,
1969b).

The Medial Geniculate Body. After lesions of the dorsal and ventral divisions
of the medial geniculate body, heavy axonal degeneration in the cortex fills the
first (AI), second (AII), posterior ectosylvian (Ep) and temporal fields of the
auditory cortex as delineated by Woolsey (1961) (Heath and Jones, 1971). The
heavy terminal degeneration in the posterior ectosylvian gyrus is confined to its
ventral two-thirds, filling only field Ep as determined by the method of evoked
potentials (Woolsey, 1961). *From the point of view of the present paper, it is important to note that, caudally, this degeneration extends only slightly into the rostral
bank of the posterior suprasylvian sulcus and stops abruptly before reaching the
fundus.* Ventrally, the degeneration in the posterior ectosylvian gyrus does not
reach as far as the rhinal sulcus, being separated by a small area a few mm wide,
which is free of degenerating fragments.

The Posterior Group. Since the posterior group of thalamic nuclei has been
shown to receive fibres from the ascending somatic and auditory pathways, its
cortical projection is also germane to the present study. Lesions involving the

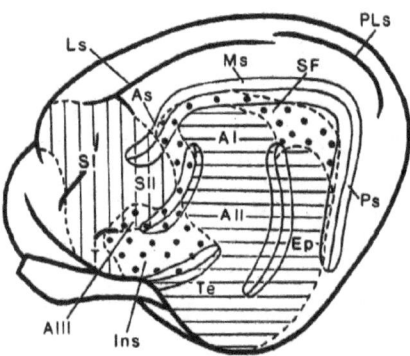

Fig. 2. A schematic diagram showing the extent of the cortex receiving fibres from the somatic (vertical hatching) and auditory (horizontal hatching) relay nuclei and from certain components of the posterior group of thalamic nuclei (dots). The ventroposterior nucleus projects to the first (*SI*) and second (*SII*) somatic sensory areas and to the taste areas (*T*). The medial geniculate body projects to all fields of the auditory cortex except the insular area (*Ins*) and suprasylvian fringe (*SF*) which receive fibres from parts of the posterior group of nuclei

suprageniculate nucleus and other adjacent parts of the posterior group (Heath and Jones, 1971) cause degeneration in a band of cortex bounding SII and most of the auditory fields. Although the band encroaches on certain parts of the suprasylvian sulcus, it does not affect the suprasylvian gyrus proper.

The band includes the insular area and extends dorsally in the banks of the anterior ectosylvian sulcus to cross the upper few mm. of the anterior ectosylvian gyrus in the suprasylvian fringe (Woolsey, 1961). It enters the vertical part of the anterior suprasylvian sulcus, filling the lateral bank and extending into the deeper half of the medial bank. It then continues caudally in the suprasylvian fringe in the lateral bank of the middle suprasylvian sulcus approximately as far as its mid point. Caudal to this mid point, it progressively comes to the surface in the dorsal one-third of the posterior ectosylvian gyrus, dorsal and caudal to AI. In the extreme postero-dorsal corner of the posterior ectosylvian gyrus, however, there is a very small area which is also free of degeneration. Otherwise, the degeneration fills the part of the gyrus lying dorsal to Ep. Caudally, the degeneration does not reach deeply into the rostral bank of the posterior suprasylvian sulcus.

The Lateral Geniculate Nucleus (Cats 40 R and 40 L). Cat 40 R shows the portions of the cortex receiving fibres from the thalamic visual relay, the dorsal lateral geniculate nucleus. The lesion is in the middle of the medio-lateral extent of the nucleus and extends throughout its caudal two-thirds (Figs. 3 and 24). It involves laminae A, A 1 and B and the central interlaminar nucleus but the medial interlaminar nucleus is definitely spared. Axonal degeneration in the cortex is confined to the lateral, postlateral and splenial gyri; it takes the form of two bands of intense terminal degeneration. In adjacent Nissl-stained sections, and even in the Nauta-stained sections themselves, it is possible to see that these two bands of degeneration are confined to areas 17 and 18. However, the common boundary between the two areas, along the crown of the lateral gyrus, contains

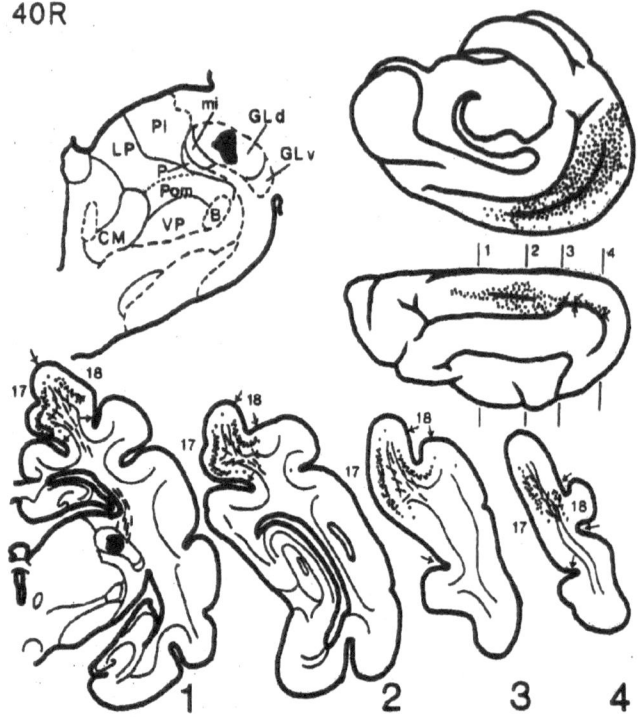

Fig. 3. The distribution of degeneration in the cortex following a lesion (black) confined to the main laminae of the dorsal lateral geniculate nucleus (see also Fig. 24). Degeneration is restricted to areas 17 and 18 of the visual cortex, the boundaries of which are indicated by small arrows on the sections. Degeneration occupies mainly the rostral parts of the two areas and is concentrated in the middle of both, conforming to the part of the retinal representation destroyed in the lateral geniculate nucleus. In this and subsequent figures terminal degeneration is indicated by stipple and degenerating fibres by short lines. Degeneration in the banks of a sulcus is indicated by arrows pointing to the appropriate bank of the sulcus

only scattered axon fragments which are inconstant from section to section and there is also relative sparing of the extreme medial part of area 17 and the extreme lateral part of area 18. The distribution of the heavy degeneration mainly to the middle portions of areas 17 and 18 conforms to the parts of the retinal representation destroyed in the lateral geniculate: in both the cortex and the lateral geniculate nucleus, there is sparing of the parts containing the representations of the vertical meridian and of the extreme periphery of the visual field.

On the opposite side of this brain, there is a second, smaller lesion in the lateral geniculate nucleus (Cat 40 L). This lesion affects the rostral half of the nucleus and is at a level medial to that in Cat 40 R (Figs. 4 and 23). It primarily affects lamina B but it encroaches upon lamina A 1 and the medial interlaminar nucleus at its rostral end. (At one point it also breaks through the optic tract and just encroaches upon

40 L

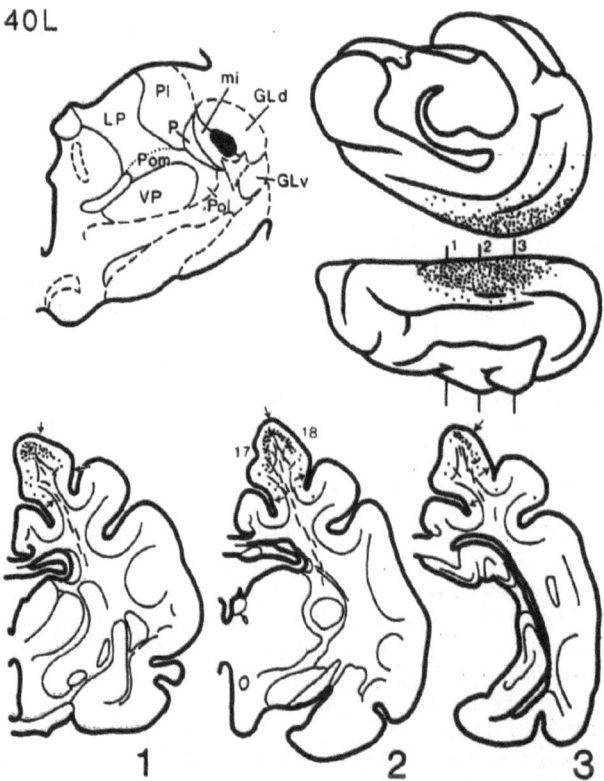

Fig. 4. An experiment in which the medial interlaminar nucleus of the lateral geniculate body was damaged in conjunction with the main laminae (see also Fig. 23). Degeneration in the visual cortex affects areas 17 and 18. Since medial parts of the nucleus were destroyed, the degeneration is concentrated in adjacent parts of the two cortical areas in which the vertical meridian of the visual field is represented. Only a very few scattered degenerating fragments were found in area 19 and in the lateral suprasylvian area (sections 2 and 3, and see text)

the dorsal division of the medial geniculate body; it is considered, Heath and Jones (1971), that this accounts for a small focus of incidental degeneration in the middle of Ep.) There is very dense terminal degeneration in the rostral halves of areas 17 and 18 but, by contrast with Cat 40R, the degenerating fragments are concentrated in the adjoining parts of the two areas where the vertical meridian is represented.

In both Cats 40L and 40R and more especially in 40L, a small number of degenerating axons are present in area 19 and in the lateral suprasylvian area. They are inconstant and are not found in all sections. Although it is not possible to exclude that this additional degeneration is due to involvement of the lateral geniculate nucleus, three facts argue against such an interpretation: it is extremely sparse; it does not conform to the retinotopic organization; fibres passing to these two additional areas from more medial parts of the thalamus, pass through the lateral geniculate nucleus *en route* (see below).

Comment

The experiments summarized in this section indicate that no parts of the middle or posterior suprasylvian gyri receive fibres directly from any sensory relay nucleus of the thalamus. Although area 19 and the lateral suprasylvian area are often considered to be a part of the primary visual cortex, the evidence militates against their receiving an input from the lateral geniculate nucleus. Thus, any sensory input to these and to other areas in the middle and posterior suprasylvian gyri must come *via* "association" nuclei such as the lateral nuclear-pulvinar complex, *via* cortico-cortical fibres from the primary sensory areas, or *via* other means. The anterior suprasylvian gyrus is obviously a part of the primary somatic sensory cortex and the remainder of the paper will be concerned with the middle and posterior suprasylvian gyri.

Cortico-Cortical Connexions from the Primary Sensory Areas

Somatic Sensory Connexions. Following lesions of SI, degenerating cortico-cortical fibres are distributed in a topographically organized fashion to the rostral parts of the lateral and middle suprasylvian gyri; the area receiving such fibres corresponds closely to the architectonic field, area 5. As this projection has been fully described in an earlier paper (Jones and Powell, 1968a), no experiments will be presented here. SII does not send fibres into the suprasylvian gyrus (Jones and Powell, 1968a).

Visual Connexions (Cats 2 and 79). Other investigations have shown that areas 17 and 18 of the visual cortex send fibres to the medial and lateral aspects of the middle suprasylvian gyrus, to areas which have been equated with area 19 and the lateral suprasylvian area (Hubel and Wiesel, 1965; Garey *et al.*, 1968; Wilson, 1968). However, the full extent of the latter areas have not been outlined on the basis of cortico-cortical connexions. In two experiments, therefore, narrow lesions were placed along the crowns of the lateral and postlateral gyri in order to destroy as much of areas 17 and 18 as were readily accessible without concomitant damage to other areas. As the distribution of degeneration in the two brains is essentially similar, only Cat 79 will be described (Fig. 5). Throughout its length, the area of damage is confined to the cortex of adjacent portions of areas 17 and 18 in which parts of the visual field adjacent to the vertical meridian are represented. Axonal degeneration outside areas 17 and 18 affects area 19 and the lateral suprasylvian area in accord with the results of the other investigations mentioned above.

Terminal degeneration outside areas 17 and 18 of the ipsilateral cortex forms two bands along the medial and lateral aspects of the middle suprasylvian gyrus. Because of the transitional nature of the cortex in the caudal parts of the gyrus and the consequent lack of clearly defined architectonic boundaries, we have not been able to correlate the margins of these bands of degeneration with obvious architectonic boundaries in Nissl stained sections. However, following the example of other investigators who have observed the dual projection from areas 17 and 18,

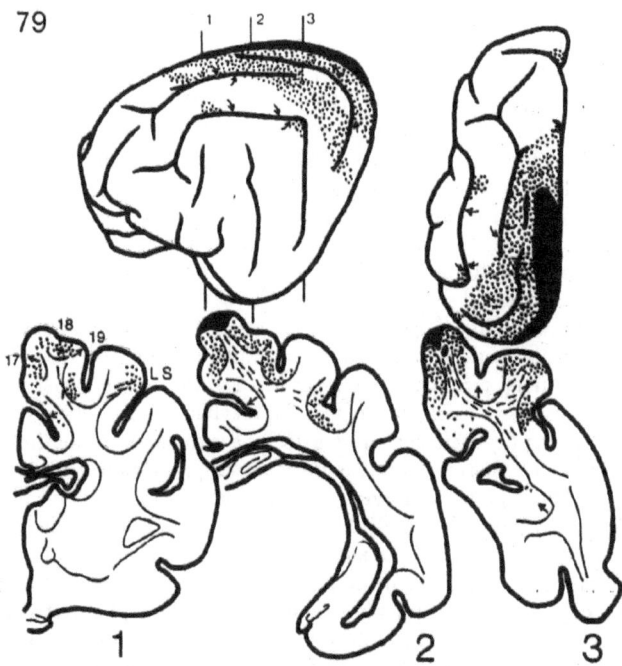

Fig. 5. The distribution of degeneration in the cortex following a large lesion of areas 17 and 18 of the visual cortex. Note the oblique lateral boundary of area 19 and the manner in which it passes close to the junction of the posterior and middle suprasylvian sulci. Note also the degeneration in the small part of area 19 lying medial to area 17 in section 1. The full extent of the lateral suprasylvian area is indicated and the manner in which it crosses from the medial to the lateral bank of the middle suprasylvian sulcus

we shall regard these two bands of degeneration as being situated in area 19 and in the lateral suprasylvian area respectively. On this basis, the lateral margin of area 19 commences in the fundus of the lateral sulcus but moves progressively into the lateral bank of the sulcus as it is followed caudally. At the caudal end of the lateral sulcus, the boundary emerges onto the surface of the middle suprasylvian gyrus and inclines ventrally and caudally, more or less parallel to the postlateral sulcus. As it crosses the junction of the middle and posterior suprasylvian gyri, this boundary passes to within a few mm. of the junction of the middle and posterior suprasylvian sulci. It then continues across the dorsal aspect of the posterior suprasylvian gyrus, passing just below the ventral end of the postlateral sulcus. Finally, it turns around the caudal surface of the hemisphere and passes on to the medial surface of the hemisphere to reach the caudal end of the splenial sulcus.

Area 19, as defined by this method occupies the fundus and lateral bank of the lateral sulcus and the postero-dorsal corners of both the middle and posterior suprasylvian gyri. The medial boundary of area 19 can be distinguished in Nissl stained sections since there is a fairly clear cytoarchitectonic change where it abuts on area 18 (Fig. 25). The most medial part of area 19 is relatively free of degenerating fragments. On the medial surface of this brain, the degeneration is limited by a line running along the fundus of the splenial sulcus. In most sections, terminal degeneration stops at the medial boundary of area 17 which lies in the upper bank of the sulcus, a little medial to the fundus. However, in the rostral half and at the extreme caudal end of the sulcus, a moderate number of degenerating fragments always extend to the fundus. According to Otsuka and Hassler (1962), this small area lying medial to area 17 is an extension of area 19 which occupies the full rostro-caudal length of the splenial sulcus. Since the degeneration in this small area is continuous across the rostral ends of the splenial and lateral gyri with that in area 19 on the lateral aspect of the hemisphere, we concur with Otsuka and Hassler. However, unlike these authors, we are unable to trace area 19 along more than the rostral half of the splenial sulcus.

On the lateral aspect of the middle suprasylvian gyrus of this brain and separated from the degeneration in area 19 by a clear area, is another region of terminal degeneration corresponding to the lateral suprasylvian area. At the rostral end of the middle suprasylvian gyrus, this degeneration fills the medial bank of the middle suprasylvian sulcus and, close to the junction of the middle and anterior suprasylvian sulci, it extends for a short distance onto the exposed surface of the middle suprasylvian gyrus. On being followed caudally, however, the degeneration on the exposed surface quickly disappears and, throughout the rest of the rostral two-thirds of the middle suprasylvian sulcus, it is confined to the medial bank. In the caudal one-third of the sulcus, the degeneration moves progressively into the lateral bank and becomes correspondingly more deeply placed in the medial bank. At the junction of the middle and posterior suprasylvian sulci, the degeneration spares the medial bank completely so that the width of the band of unaffected cortex separating it from the degeneration in area 19 is maintained. It fills the lateral bank and encroaches on the extreme postero-dorsal corner of the posterior ectosylvian gyrus, barely entering the upper part of the posterior suprasylvian sulcus.

The distribution of *commissural degeneration* in the opposite cortex of this brain supports the delimitation of the lateral suprasylvian area indicated by the distribution of degenerating axons on the ipsilateral side. Degenerating commissural fibres distribute terminal degeneration to a band of cortex in the banks of the contralateral middle suprasylvian sulcus exactly as on the ipsilateral side. The band encroaches on the exposed surface of the middle suprasylvian gyrus rostrally; caudally, it stops in the upper part of the rostral bank of the posterior suprasylvian sulcus. Degeneration fills the medio-lateral extent of the band of cortex so that all parts of the opposite lateral suprasylvian area receive degenerating commissural fibres. Elsewhere in the opposite cortex, degeneration is confined to the parts of areas 17 and 18 adjoining their common boundary in the lateral and post-lateral gyri (Garey et al., 1968; Wilson, 1968).

Auditory Connexions (Cats 3, 59, 61 and 64). Experiments with lesions restricted to each of the several fields of the auditory cortex in the sylvian and ecto-sylvian gyri, show that none send fibres into the middle suprasylvian gyrus (Fig. 6). With the exception of the insular and temporal fields, however, all send

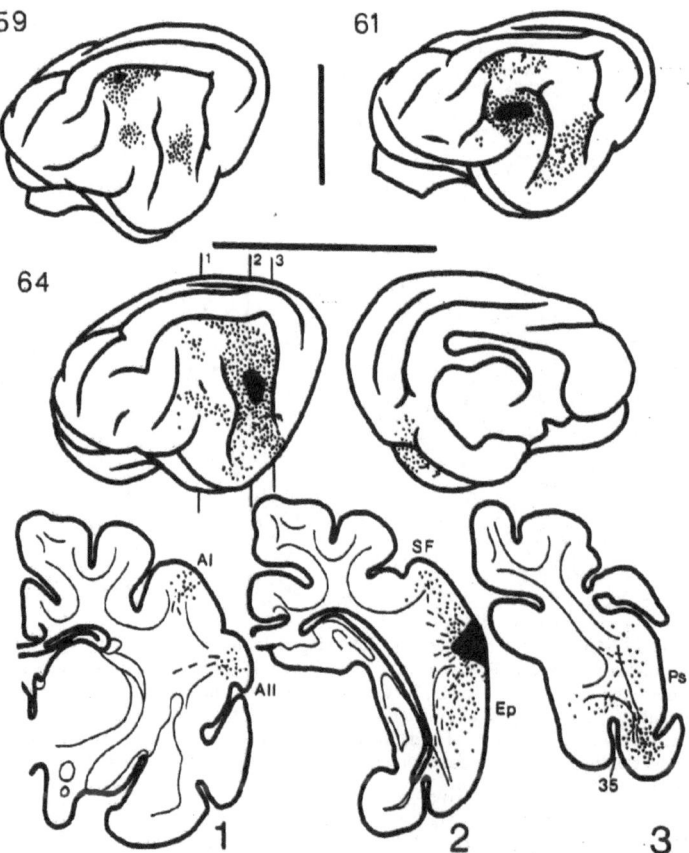

Fig. 6. Three experiments in which parts of areas *AI* (Cat 59), *AII* (Cat 61) and *Ep* (Cat 64) of the auditory cortex were destroyed. Each lesion causes degeneration in topographically related parts of the other two areas and in the suprasylvian fringe. In addition, in Cat 64, degeneration spreads into the fundus of the posterior suprasylvian sulcus (*Ps*) and into the peri-rhinal area (area 35). The sections are from Cat 64 only

fibres in an organized manner, to the suprasylvian fringe and one, Ep, has a projection to the cortex in the fundus of the posterior suprasylvian sulcus. The insular area sends fibres only to the frontal cortex and the temporal area to both the frontal cortex and to the caudal end of the cingulate gyrus.

Field Ep (Cats 3 and 64). In both of these brains there are lesions in the middle of Ep (Fig. 6). These cause terminal degeneration in topographically related parts (mainly the basal cochlear representation) of fields AI, AII and the suprasylvian fringe. There is terminal degeneration throughout Ep. The degeneration at the lower end of Ep spreads caudally into the fundus and posterior bank of the posterior suprasylvian sulcus but it does not reach the exposed surface of the

62

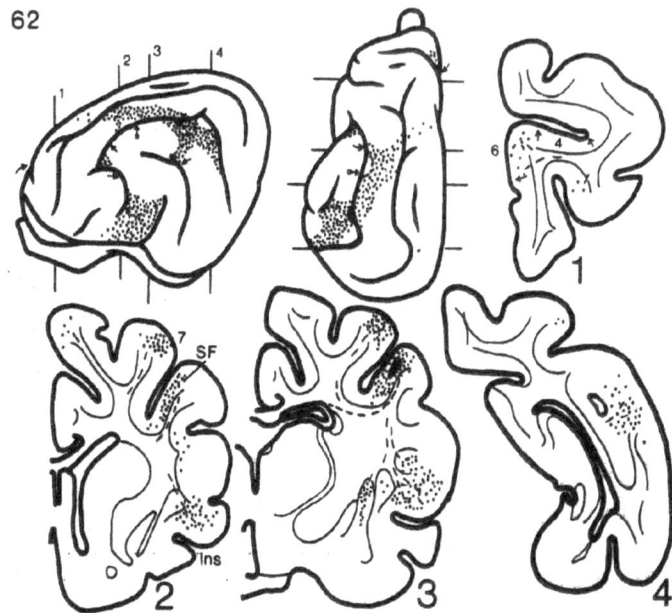

Fig. 7. The distribution of degeneration following a lesion of the suprasylvian fringe. The position of the lesion is indicated by the ringed arrows. This causes terminal degeneration throughout the suprasylvian fringe, in the insular cortex and in area 7 of the suprasylvian and lateral gyri, together with a few fragments in area 6 of the frontal lobe. Note the triangular shape of area 7 and, at its rostral end, the small bare patch close to the suprasylvian sulcus. This is the small part of the lateral suprasylvian visual area which comes to the surface at that point

posterior suprasylvian gyrus. From the sulcus, and below the lesion, degeneration reaches to the fundus of the rhinal sulcus, extending rostrally as a narrow band in this position almost to the level of the pseudosylvian sulcus. This degeneration is in the peri-rhinal area (area 35 of Gurewitsch and Chatschaturian, 1928). It should be noted that when lesions of the other auditory fields such as are shown in Fig. 6 cause degeneration in Ep, the degeneration does not reach into the rhinal and posterior suprasylvian sulci.

The Suprasylvian Fringe (Cat 62). Because the suprasylvian fringe at its caudal end comes to the surface of the posterior ectosylvian gyrus, it is possible to damage it selectively by thrusting a needle through the exposed portion and along the lateral bank of the middle suprasylvian sulcus. This was done in experiment 62 (Fig. 7). The needle track, which is confined to the cortex, enters the suprasylvian fringe in the upper part of the posterior ectosylvian gyrus and runs along the superficial half of the lateral bank of the sulcus to about its mid point. There is heavy terminal degeneration throughout the undamaged parts of the fringe conforming to the boundaries of this area defined by the distribution of degenerating thalamo-cortical fibres in experiments involving the posterior group

(Fig. 2). There are three additional areas of heavy terminal degeneration in the ipsilateral cortex. One of these is the insular area and the degeneration in it is continuous through the banks of the anterior ectosylvian sulcus and across the upper part of the anterior extosylvian gyrus with that in the suprasylvian fringe.

The second focus of terminal degeneration is mainly in the middle suprasylvian gyrus, in what will be identified as area 7. The degeneration fills a triangular area occupying the rostral and lateral aspects of the gyrus. At its rostral end (the base of the triangle) where it abuts on area 5, it fills the full width of the gyrus and a narrow band of fragments extends medially through the lateral sulcus and lateral gyrus as far as the rostral extremity of the splenial sulcus on the medial aspect of the hemisphere. In the middle suprasylvian gyrus, the area of degeneration tapers caudally to an apex situated on the medial bank of the middle suprasylvian sulcus close to its junction with the posterior suprasylvian sulcus.

A striking feature of the degeneration in this brain is the manner in which it fills the suprasylvian fringe and the triangular area 7 dorsal to it, but spares the lateral suprasylvian area lying between them. In other words, the lateral border of area 7 is coextensive with the medial border of the lateral suprasylvian area. Apparently because of this common boundary, at the rostral end of the middle suprasylvian gyrus, the small portion of the lateral suprasylvian area which comes to the surface there forms a degeneration-free patch invaginating the heavy degeneration in area 7. Just in front of this, the degeneration in area 7 and in the suprasylvian fringe becomes continuous through the banks of the dorsal part of the anterior suprasylvian sulcus.

A slight architectonic change can be detected at the junction of area 7 and the lateral suprasylvian area but at the medial boundary of area 7 there is no clear-cut boundary which may be correlated in Nissl-stained sections with the edge of the degeneration filled area in adjoining Nauta-stained sections. However, from a comparison of experiments 79 and 2 with 62 it is probable that in its rostral part the boundary lies between areas 7 and 19. More caudally, when comparing experiments 2, 79 and 62 with one another and with experiments 23 and 71 (below), there appears to be a narrow additional area intercalated between the two.

The remaining patch of terminal degeneration in the ipsilateral cortex of this brain occupies most of area 6aβ of Hassler and Muhs-Clement (1964), extending as a narrow band from the lateral bank of the presylvian sulcus, across the anterior sigmoid gyrus into the antero-medial aspect of the ventral bank of the cruciate sulcus and reappearing on the medial surface of the hemisphere (Fig. 7).

The degeneration of commissural fibres in the opposite cortex will not be illustrated but it may be noted that it is confined to the suprasylvian fringe.

Comment

These experiments show that each of the primary sensory areas are related to discrete fields in the suprasylvian gyrus: SI sends fibres to area 5; the visual areas, 17 and 18, to area 19 and to the lateral suprasylvian area; certain of the auditory fields to the suprasylvian fringe, which then projects to area 7. In addition, field Ep of the auditory cortex has a projection to the fundus of the posterior suprasylvian sulcus, to a region which extends medially in to the perirhinal cortex.

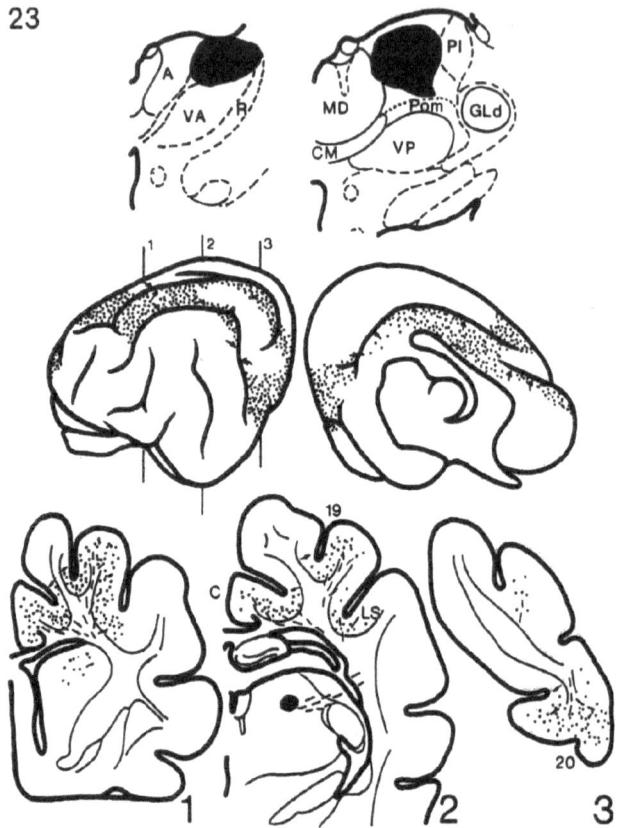

Fig. 8. The distribution of degeneration in the cortex following a large lesion affecting the lateralis dorsalis, lateralis posterior, posterior and anterior nuclei of the thalamus with smaller amounts of damage to the medio-dorsal nucleus and pulvinar. The cortical degeneration affects area 19 and the lateral suprasylvian area at the medial and lateral margins of the suprasylvian gyrus, areas 5 and 7 of the middle suprasylvian gyrus and area 20 at the ventral end of the posterior suprasylvian gyrus. Note the bare area at the junction of the middle and posterior suprasylvian gyri. Other degeneration is found in the frontal lobe and in the cingulate gyrus (*C*). The medial boundaries of areas 17 and 19 are indicated by arrows

Thalamic Connexions of the Areas in the Suprasylvian Gyrus

The individuality of areas 5, 7, 19 and the lateral suprasylvian area shown on the basis of cortico-cortical connexions, may be further brought out by a study of their thalamic connexions. Even with the horizontal stereotaxic approach, the relevant parts of the thalamus are difficult to destroy without concomitant damage of adjacent nuclei or interruption of thalamo-cortical fibres leaving them. We shall attempt to overcome this problem, first, by correlating the results of a number of experiments with large lesions of the thalamus and, second, by comparing these with the results of experiments with lesions of relevant cortical areas. The latter show the distribution of cortico-thalamic fibres which generally, though not invariably, reciprocate the thalamo-cortical connexions. The experiments presented in the first section of these results showed that the thalamo-cortical input to the suprasylvian gyrus is to be sought among thalamic nuclei other than the sensory relay nuclei, or the posterior group system of nuclei. A priori, therefore, and from earlier retrograde cell degeneration studies (Waller and Barris, 1937), the lateral nuclear complex and pulvinar are the most likely to be involved.

Cat 23. The greater part of the thalamic input to the gyrus is demonstrated by experiment 23 in which a large lesion destroys the rostral three-quarters of the nucleus lateralis posterior (Fig. 8). At its caudal end, the lesion encroaches on the posterior nucleus (of Rioch, 1929) and the ventral aspect of the pulvinar but most of the latter escapes damage. At its rostral end, the lesion destroys most of the nucleus lateralis dorsalis and invades adjacent portions of the central lateral, medio-dorsal and anterior nuclei.

Terminal degeneration occupies the parts of the suprasylvian gyrus which have been defined above as areas 5, 7, 19 and the lateral suprasylvian area, together with the fundus of the posterior suprasylvian sulcus and a small triangular area at the ventral end of the posterior suprasylvian gyrus. Degeneration spreads from the cingulate gyrus across the rostral ends of the lateral and middle suprasylvian gyri. The whole middle suprasylvian gyrus contains dense terminal degeneration from the fundus of the lateral sulcus medially, to that of the middle suprasylvian sulcus laterally. Its rostral limit is the line of junction between area 5 and SI, along the caudal bank of the ansate sulcus. As it is followed caudally, the degeneration splits into two streams, one running in area 19 and following it across the caudal surface of the brain; the other is laterally placed and appears to lie within area 7 and the lateral suprasylvian area, for it sinks progressively into the middle suprasylvian sulcus. The medial bank of the sulcus remains filled with degenerating fragments to its junction with the posterior suprasylvian sulcus. The degeneration then crosses the postero-dorsal corner of the posterior ectosylvian gyrus and enters the posterior suprasylvian sulcus. It descends, first in the rostral and then in the caudal bank of the sulcus, to emerge on the surface of the ventral part of the posterior suprasylvian gyrus. Here, there is a small triangular area of terminal degeneration extending as far medially as the rhinal sulcus. This area has previously (Heath and Jones, 1970) been equated with area 20 of the primate brain. There is a definite change in the character of the degeneration as one passes into area 20. The coarse fibre and terminal degeneration in the lateral suprasylvian area and in the fundus of the posterior suprasylvian sulcus are replaced by very much finer, and somewhat less intense axonal and terminal degeneration. As area 20 is followed on to the caudal and medial surfaces of the hemisphere, the degeneration in it becomes continuous with that in area 19, but the junction can be discerned here, also, because of similar differences in the nature of the degeneration in the two areas (Figs. 26 and 27).

Of special interest in this brain is a narrow band of degeneration-free cortex running obliquely across the upper half of the posterior suprasylvian gyrus parallel to, and separating the degeneration in area 19 from that in the posterior suprasylvian sulcus and, more rostrally, from that in area 7. This band is almost identical

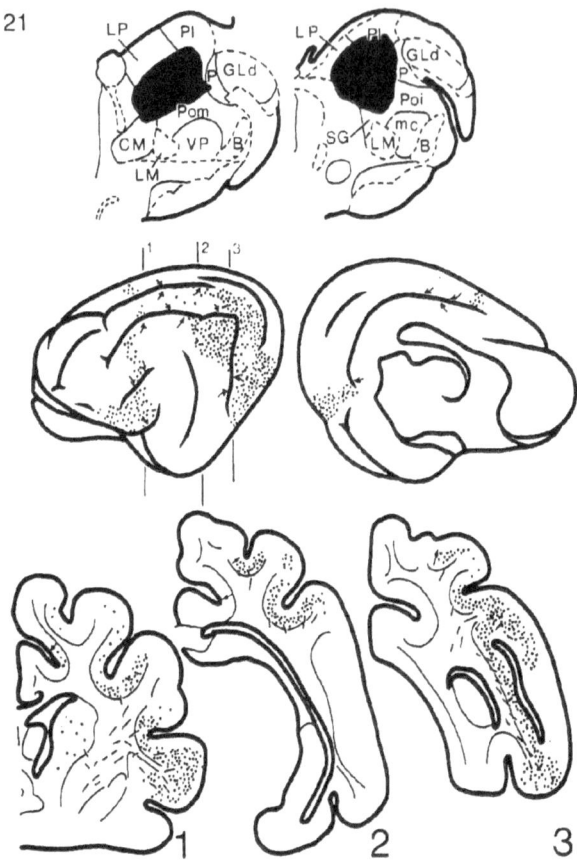

Fig. 9. A large lesion affecting mainly caudal parts of the n. lateralis posterior, together which the posterior nucleus and much of the pulvinar. The posterior group is also affected. Degeneration is found in area 19 and the lateral suprasylvian area and in most of the posterior suprasylvian gyrus, but rostral parts of the middle suprasylvian gyrus are largely free. Note how the degeneration in the suprasylvian gyrus forms a complementary pattern to that in the preceding experiment (Fig. 8) in which less of the pulvinar was damaged. Note also how the degeneration in area 19 forms a C-shaped band encircling areas 17 and 18 except in the caudal half of the splenial sulcus. Degeneration in the insular cortex and suprasylvian fringe is due to involvement by the lesion of the posterior group

with that mentioned in Cat 62 as probably separating the caudal part of area 7 from area 19 (Fig. 7).

Terminal degeneration observed in the ventral bank of the cruciate sulcus (area 6) and in the cingulate gyrus of this brain is assumed to be due to damage of the medio-dorsal and anterior nuclei and will not be described in detail. The degeneration in the cingulate gyrus extends to the fundus of the splenial sulcus and abuts on the medial boundary of area 17 throughout the length of the sulcus. It appears to occupy the anterior limbic, cingulate and retrosplenial areas (Rose and Woolsey, 1948 b) as well as the small part of area 19 situated in the rostral half of, and at the caudal end of the splenial sulcus.

Cat 21. The degeneration-free area seen in the posterior suprasylvian gyrus of the preceding experiment becomes filled with terminal degeneration in an experiment (Cat 21) in which more of the pulvinar is damaged (Fig. 9). In this brain, the lesion destroys the caudal half of the nucleus lateralis posterior with the suprageniculate nucleus and other parts of the posterior group. It extends dorsally and laterally to destroy the caudal two-thirds of the pulvinar and adjacent parts of the posterior nucleus. There is a small medial extension into the medio-dorsal nucleus.

In the cortex of this brain there are two bands of terminal degeneration which converge on the posterior suprasylvian gyrus. One commences at the middle of the antero-posterior extent of the splenial sulcus, in the small part of area 19 adjoining area 17. This continues forwards in the depths of the sulcus, then it passes dorsally and laterally across the rostral ends of the splenial and lateral gyri, approximately 1 cm. behind the ansate sulcus, to enter the fundus and lateral bank of the lateral sulcus. In this position, it continues caudally, obviously in area 19, and, turning across the caudal surface of the hemisphere, it ends in the caudal few mm. of the splenial sulcus. As this degeneration in area 19 crosses the junction of the middle and posterior suprasylvian gyri, it progressively expands laterally beyond the boundary of area 19 as defined in Cat 79, and is joined by degeneration in the lateral suprasylvian area and in the suprasylvian fringe extending caudally from these into the posterior suprasylvian sulcus. The posterior suprasylvian gyrus is filled with terminal degeneration although the degeneration is less intense just posterior to the upper half of the posterior suprasylvian sulcus (Fig. 9). Ventrally, the degeneration in the posterior suprasylvian gyrus extends as far as the lateral bank of the rhinal sulcus and in this position, extends forwards ventral to field Ep of the auditory cortex. There are a few scattered axon fragments on the crown of the middle suprasylvian gyrus (in area 7) but, on the whole, the degeneration forms a complementary pattern to that seen in the preceding experiment in which mainly rostral parts of the lateral nuclear complex and only at little of the pulvinar were damaged. It suggests that the small area left free in the preceding experiment receives thalamo-cortical fibres from the pulvinar.

Elsewhere in the cortex of Cat 21, the insular area, suprasylvian fringe and lateral suprasylvsian area are filled with terminal degeneration and parts of the orbito-frontal cortex are also affected. There is a small amount of terminal degeneration in the basolateral nuclei of the amygdala in both cats 23 and 21.

Cat 20 (not illustrated). In this brain, a lesion mainly of the ventromedial aspect of the lateralis posterior and of the suprageniculate nuclei but with extensions into the ventral part of the pulvinar, central lateral and medio-dorsal nuclei, causes degeneration mainly in area 5 of the middle suprasylvian gyrus. Additional heavy degeneration is present in the suprasylvian fringe, lateral suprasylvian area, insular cortex, area 20, and in parts of the orbito-frontal cortex. A few degenerating fibres reach the amygdala.

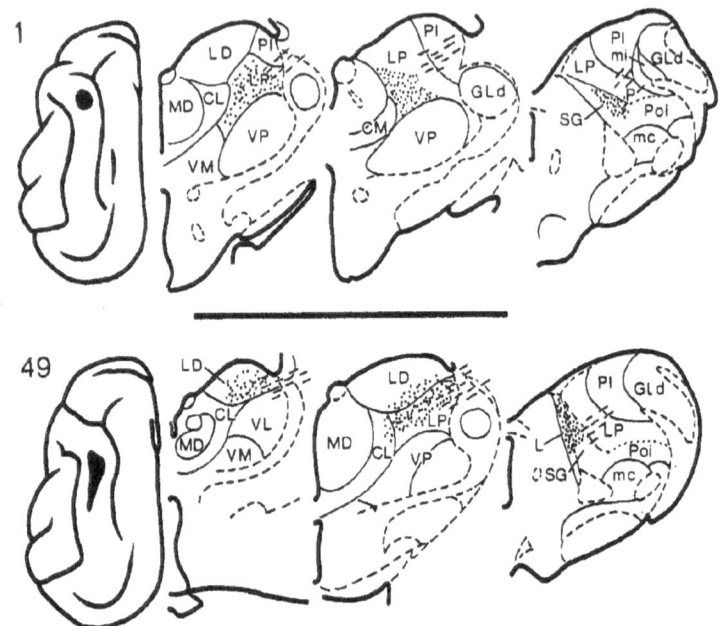

Fig. 10. Showing the distribution of cortico-thalamic fibres in two brains in which areas 5 (Cat 1) and 7 (Cat 49) were damaged. In Cat 1, terminal degeneration affects the rostral and ventro-medial aspects of the n. lateralis posterior and the lateral aspect of the suprageniculate nucleus. In Cat 49, it affects the n. lateralis dorsalis, rostral and dorsal aspects of the n. lateralis posterior and medial parts of the suprageniculate nucleus and n. limitans. A small number of fragments are also seen in the central lateral nucleus in Cat 49

Cortico-Thalamic Connexions. Lesions have been placed in most of the cortical areas defined in earlier sections of these results. In all of the experiments involving lesions of the middle and posterior suprasylvian gyri, terminal degeneration is found in three nuclei of the thalamus: in a part of the lateral nuclear complex or pulvinar; in a part of the intralaminar-posterior group system of nuclei (Jones and Powell, 1971); and in a part of the reticular nucleus.

Area 5 (Cat 1). Following a lesion confined to area 5 in the rostral end of the middle suprasylvian gyrus (Fig. 10), terminal degeneration is found in the rostral and ventro-medial aspect of the nucleus lateralis posterior. Other degeneration is present in the dorsal and lateral aspect of the suprageniculate nucleus and in a small part of the reticular nucleus near the rostral pole of the lateral geniculate nucleus.

Area 7 (Cat 49). A lesion situated in area 7 (Fig. 10) causes degeneration of cortico-thalamic fibres and terminals in the whole nucleus lateralis dorsalis and this extends caudally into the rostral and dorsal aspects of the nucleus lateralis posterior. Other degeneration is present in the dorso-lateral aspect of the central lateral nucleus, in the most medial aspect of the suprageniculate nucleus and the

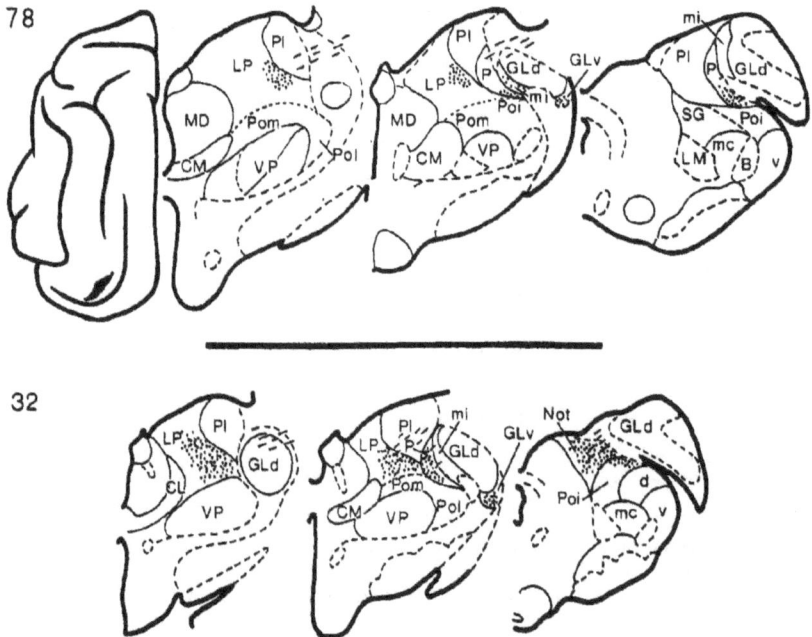

Fig. 11. The distribution of degenerating cortico-thalamic fibres in two brains in which parts of area 19 (Cat 78) and the lateral suprasylvian area (Cat 32) were damaged. In both, there is degeneration in essentially the same parts of the n. lateralis posterior and in the posterior and the ventral lateral geniculate nuclei. In addition, the lesion of area 19 causes degeneration in the medial interlaminar nucleus and that of the lateral suprasylvian area in the nucleus of the optic tract and in the most caudal part of the posterior group

adjoining nucleus limitans, as well as in a part of the reticular nucleus lying dorsal to the lateral geniculate nucleus.

Area 19 (Cat 78). A small lesion of area 19 on the exposed surface of the caudal part of the middle suprasylvian gyrus, close to the postlateral sulcus (Figs. 11 and 25), causes dense terminal degeneration (Fig. 28) in the ventro-lateral aspect of the nucleus lateralis posterior over the middle portion of its rostrocaudal extent, and terminal fragments are also found in the adjacent posterior nucleus and in the medial interlaminar nucleus of the lateral geniculate body. No degeneration is present in the main laminae of the dorsal lateral geniculate nucleus but a small focus of coarse degeneration is seen in the middle of the ventral lateral geniculate nucleus. Other terminal degeneration is present in the nucleus of the optic tract and in the pretectum. The lesion of areas 17 and 18 described above (Cat 79, Fig. 5) results in terminal degeneration in the lateral half of the nucleus lateralis posterior, and in the main laminae of the lateral geniculate nucleus but in none of the other nuclei of the thalamus showing degeneration after the lesion of area 19.

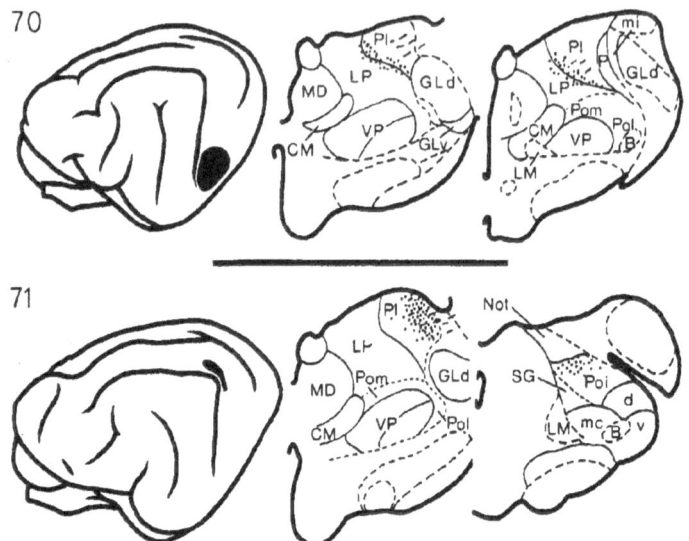

Fig. 12. Experiments with lesions of the dorsal and ventral (area 20) aspects of the posterior suprasylvian gyrus. Each causes degeneration of cortico-thalamic fibres in different parts of the pulvinar and in the intermediate divisions of the posterior group

The Lateral Suprasylvian Area (Cats 16 and 32). Because the lateral suprasylvian area comes to the surface at its rostral end, it may be damaged selectively by thrusting a needle through the exposed portion and along the medial bank of the middle suprasylvian sulcus. This was done in two experiments (Cats 16 and 32) (Fig. 11). In both, there is terminal degeneration throughout the lateral half of the nucleus lateralis posterior, in approximately the same region as after lesions of the other three visual areas. Additional heavy degeneration is present in the posterior nucleus and in the medial half of the ventral lateral geniculate nucleus as well as in the pretectum, nucleus of the optic tract and in the most caudal part of the posterior group lying adjacent to the latter. There is no degeneration in the dorsal lateral geniculate nucleus. Degeneration in the reticular nucleus is confined to the vicinity of the lateral geniculate body.

The Upper Part of the Posterior Suprasylvian Gyrus (Cats 46 and 71). In these two brains the lesion is at the junction of the middle and posterior suprasylvian gyri and in both the distribution of degeneration in the cortex (see below) suggests that it is restricted to the narrow area which separates areas 7 and 19. In the ipsilateral thalamus of both brains, there is a focus of terminal degeneration throughout most of the pulvinar but more particularly in its lateral half (Fig. 12). The degeneration is relatively sparse and is made up of very fine fibres and terminals (Fig. 29).

Area 20 (Cats 10, 68 and 70). In these three brains, there are lesions which, as far as one can tell in the absence of clear-cut architectonic boundaries in the region, are confined to area 20. In all of them there is relatively sparse and extremely fine degeneration in a strip running along the border between the pulvinar and the nucleus lateralis posterior (Fig. 12). It seems to involve mainly the pulvinar but it cannot be excluded that the lateralis posterior is also affected.

Comment

On the basis of cortico-thalamic connexions, the various areas defined in the earlier parts of these results are obviously related to different parts of the lateral nuclear complex or pulvinar. Although there is a considerable overlap, especially in the rostral part of the lateralis posterior, the following pattern appears to hold: area 19 and the lateral suprasylvian area send fibres to the posterior nucleus and to the lateral half of the lateralis posterior, overlapping projections from areas 17 and/or 18 to the latter; area 5 sends fibres to the ventro-medial quadrant of the lateralis posterior; area 7 to the lateralis dorsalis and the rostral and dorsal aspects of the lateralis posterior; area 20 to the ventro-medial aspect of the pulvinar; the strip of cortex separating areas 7 and 19 sends fibres to most of the remainder of the pulvinar.

This pattern may by compared with the results of experiments involving stereotaxic lesions in the thalamus. A lesion affecting the lateralis dorsalis, the rostral part of the lateralis posterior, the posterior nucleus and the ventral aspect of the pulvinar (Cat 23, Fig. 8) caused degeneration in areas 5, 7, 19, 20 and the lateral suprasylvian area. A small lesion mainly of the ventro-medial part of the lateralis posterior (Cat 20) caused degeneration in area 5 and in the rostral parts of area 19 and the lateral suprasylvian area. A lesion of the caudal part of the lateralis posterior, posterior nucleus and most of the pulvinar (Cat 21 R, Fig. 9), on the other hand, caused degeneration of thalamo-cortical fibres in areas 19 and 20, in the lateral suprasylvian area and in the strip of cortex separating the caudal parts of areas 7 and 19 from one another, with a few scattered fragments in area 7. In all of these brains, therefore, the relationship between the various areas of the suprasylvian gyrus and the lateral nuclear-pulvinar complex appears to be confirmed by the two different approaches.

Cortico-Cortical connexions within the Suprasylvian Gyrus

By studying the distribution of degenerating cortico-cortical fibres following lesions of the various fields of the suprasylvian gyrus, an indication can be given of the inter-relationships of these fields and of the sequence of association connexions proceeding outwards from the primary sensory areas. Already, it has been shown that: SI sends fibres to area 5; the suprasylvian fringe to area 7; Ep to the fundus of the posterior suprasylvian sulcus and the peri-rhinal area; areas 17 and/or 18 to area 19 and to the lateral suprasylvian area.

Area 5 (Cat 1). The part of area 5 situated at the rostral end of the middle suprasylvian gyrus was damaged in Cat 1 and Nissl-stained sections show that the area of damage is confined to area 5 (Fig. 13). A continuous band of terminal degeneration spreads through the undamaged parts of area 5 and back into area 7. The rostral limit of this band of degeneration is a line commencing in the medial bank of the vertical limb of the anterior suprasylvian sulcus and extending across

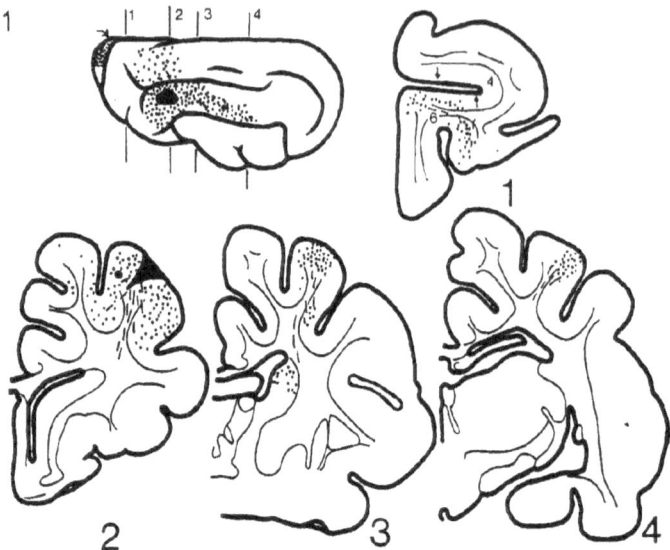

Fig. 13. An experiment in which a lesion of area 5 causes terminal degeneration in area 7 of the suprasylvian gyrus and in area 6 of the frontal cortex

the suprasylvian and lateral gyri approximately along the line of the fundus of the ansate sulcus, to reach the medial surface of the hemisphere and terminate at the rostral extremity of the splenial sulcus. The rostro-caudal extent of this band of degeneration is very narrow in the lateral and splenial gyri but, on passing through the lateral sulcus and into the middle suprasylvian gyrus, it expands rapidly in a caudal direction. The medial margin of the band of degeneration follows the oblique medial boundary defined for area 7 in Cats 62 and 23, so that the degeneration tapers to an apex near the junction of the middle and posterior suprasylvian sulci. The lateral boundary follows the boundary of area 7 along the lip of the middle suprasylvian sulcus, sinking into the medial bank of the sulcus caudally. At its rostral end, the small portion of the lateral suprasylvian area which comes to the surface of the middle suprasylvian gyrus again stands out by being free of degeneration. In front of it, the degeneration in areas 5 and 7 reaches to the middle of the rostral bank of the anterior suprasylvian sulcus.

There is a small amount of degeneration in the frontal lobe. This lies within area 6aβ of Hassler and Muhs-Clement (1964) extending across the medial aspect of the anterior sigmoid gyrus and into the medial part of the ventral bank of the cruciate sulcus.

Area 7 (Cat 49). In this cat, the lesion is in the part of area 7 situated at the rostral end of the middle suprasylvian gyrus (Fig. 14) and terminal degeneration spreads medially and laterally to fill the remainder of area 7 lying here, but again sparing the small exposed part of the lateral suprasylvian area. In front of the lesion, terminal degeneration reaches to the region of the suprasylvian fringe

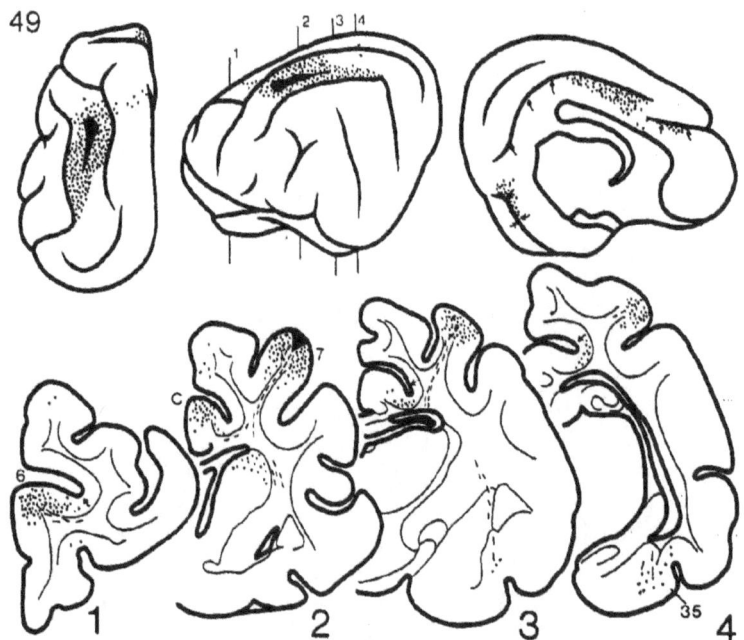

49

Fig. 14. The distribution of degeneration in the cortex following a lesion of area 7. Note how this defines the triangular shape of area 7; note also the additional foci of degeneration in the cingulate area (*C*), the peri-rhinal area (area 35) and the frontal lobe (area 6)

in the rostral bank of the anterior suprasylvian sulcus. A narrow strip of terminal degeneration also spreads medially across the lateral gyrus to the rostral end of the splenial sulcus. As the degeneration in the middle suprasylvian gyrus is followed caudally, it narrows to an apex near the junction of the middle and posterior suprasylvian sulci, as in the preceding experiment. Area 7 is, thus, filled with degenerating axons and terminals.

There are three other areas of dense terminal degeneration in the ipsilateral cortex of this brain. In the frontal lobe, the whole ventral bank of the cruciate sulcus is filled with fragments and these spread on to the medial and rostral surfaces of the hemisphere, so that virtually all three subfields of area 6 of Hassler and Muhs-Clement (1964) are filled. The second area of terminal degeneration is on the medial surface of the brain and commences by filling the cortex covering the rostral one-third of the cingulate gyrus. When traced caudally, however, it rapidly narrows and becomes a strip situated in the ventral bank of the splenial sulcus and coming in contact with the medial boundary of area 17 in the middle part of the sulcus. In the rostral part of the sulcus, it is separated by a narrow strip of normal cortex from the boundary of area 17. The third isolated patch of dense terminal degeneration is quite small and is situated in the fundus and medial bank of the caudal half of the rhinal sulcus, in the peri-rhinal cortex (area 35).

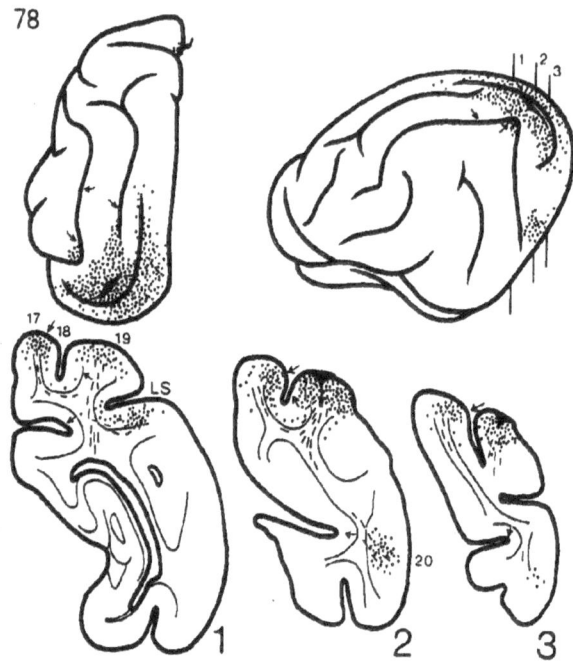

Fig. 15. The distribution of degeneration in the cortex following a small lesion confined to area 19 (see also Fig. 25). The degeneration affects the caudal parts of areas 17, 18 and 19; in areas 17 and 18 it is restricted to the representation of the vertical meridian. Other foci of degeneration appear in the caudal part of the lateral suprasylvian area and in area 20 A few additional fragments are found in area 6

Area 19 (Cat 78). The efferent cortico-cortical connexions of area 19 are shown by the experiment, described in the preceding section, in which there is a relatively small lesion confined to this area near the postlateral sulcus (Fig. 15). It results in terminal degeneration: in the caudal halves of areas 17 and 18 and especially at the boundary between the two; in the part of the lateral suprasylvian area situated in the caudal half of the middle suprasylvian sulcus and extending on to the upper part of the posterior ectosylvian gyrus; in area 20 at the ventral end of the posterior suprasylvian gyrus; in the frontal lobe at the antero-medial end of the ventral bank of the cruciate sulcus. In area 19 itself, the terminal degeneration fills it from approximately the level of overlap of the lateral and postlateral sulci across the caudal surface of the hemisphere and into the caudal end of the splenial sulcus.

Cat 12. In order to show the full extent of the efferent cortical connexions of area 19, reference may be made to Cat 12 in which a greater proportion of area 19 was damaged, although in conjunction with areas 17 and 18 (Fig. 16). This experiment must, therefore, be controlled by reference to cats 78 and 79 (Figs. 5 and 15).

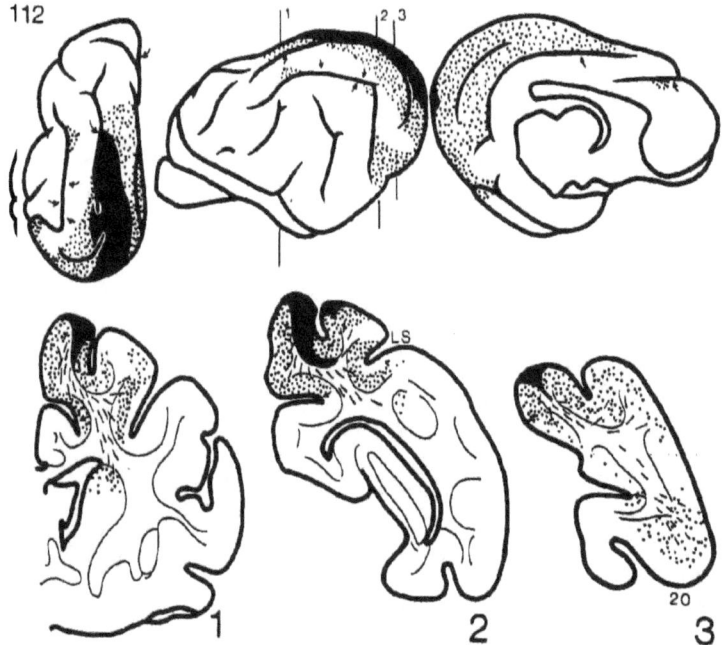

Fig. 16. An experiment in which the distribution of terminal degeneration following a large lesion of areas 17, 18 and 19 defines the full extent of areas 19 and 20 and of the lateral suprasylvian area. Note how in the rostral part of the splenial sulcus (section 1) degeneration extends beyond the medial boundary of area 17 (small arrow) into the small part of area 19 situated there. Note also how the lateral suprasylvian area comes to the surface at its rostral and caudal ends

The lesion destroys the crowns of the lateral and postlateral gyri and undercuts a good deal of the medial bank of the lateral and postlateral sulci so as to affect area 19.

Lateral to the lesion, degeneration spreads to the boundary of area 19 defined in cats 2 and 79. Most of the crown of the middle suprasylvian gyrus is free of degeneration; then, lateral to this, there is again heavy degeneration throughont the full length of the lateral suprasylvian area. Although this degeneration encroaches on the rostral bank of the posterior suprasylvian sulcus, the upper half of the sulcus is otherwise free of degeneration. The lower half of the caudal bank, however, contains a narrow band of fine but heavy terminal degeneration which expands caudally onto the lower part of the exposed surface of the posterior suprasylvian gyrus to reach area 19 caudally and the rhinal sulcus ventrally. This corresponds to area 20 as defined in Cat 23 (Fig. 8). The upper half of the posterior suprasylvian gyrus is free of degeneration and there is, again, a narrow strip of cortex separating the heavy degeneration in area 19 from that in the lateral suprasylvian area at the junction of the middle and posterior suprasylvian sulci. In the frontal lobe, most of area 6aβ is filled with sparse terminal degeneration.

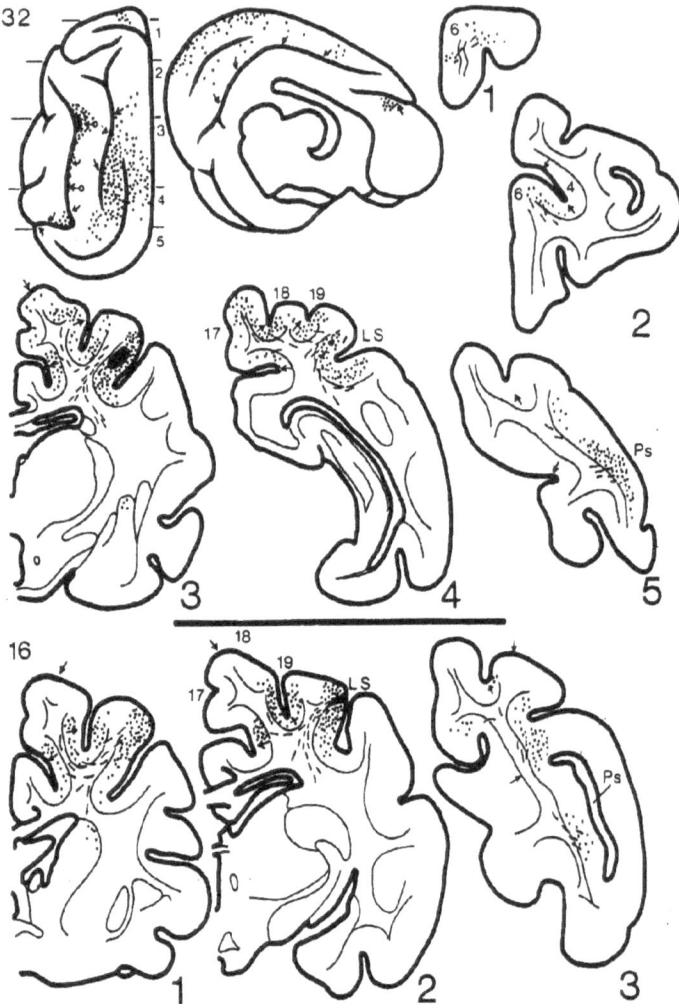

Fig. 17. Two experiments in which parts of the lateral suprasylvian area were destroyed. In cat 16 (lower), a lesion along the medial margin of the lateral suprasylvian area causes degeneration in those parts of areas 17, 18 and 19 representing the periphery of the visual field, in the fundus of the posterior suprasylvian sulcus (*Ps*) and in area 6 of the frontal lobe. In cat 32 (upper) a larger lesion causes much more extensive degeneration in areas 17, 18 and 19. Note how in the rostral end of the splenial sulcus (section 3) degeneration affects the small part of area 19 lying medial to area 17

The Lateral Suprasylvian Area (Cats 16 and 32). The two experiments in which the lateral suprasylvian area was damaged (Fig. 17) show the efferent cortical connexions of this area. The smaller lesion is in Cat 16 and, entering the exposed part of the area at the rostral end of the middle suprasylvian gyrus, it extends along the medial bank of the middle suprasylvian sulcus just beneath the surface. The lesion in Cat 32 has a similar entry point but is larger and becomes progressively more deeply placed as it is followed caudally. It destroys the cortex in the superficial half of the medial bank of the sulcus, approximately between the levels of the anterior and posterior ectosylvian sulci; at one point a few petechial haemorrhages affect the fundus of the sulcus also. Experiment 16, in affecting the most medial part of the lateral suprasylvian area, would damage mostly the representation of the periphery of the retina (Hubel and Wiesel, 1969). A far greater proportion of the total representation would be affected in Cat 32.

In Cat 32, those parts of the lateral suprasylvian area not damaged by the lesion are filled with heavy terminal degeneration. Apart from a localized area around the entry point of the needle, no degeneration extends onto the exposed surface of the middle suprasylvian gyrus. At the caudal end of the middle suprasylvian sulcus, the degeneration in the lateral suprasylvian area becomes less and appears about to cease but, on turning into the fundus of the posterior suprasylvian sulcus, it abruptly becomes more intense and continues along the fundus of the sulcus to its lower end, encroaching a little on the caudal bank adjacent to area 20. The region of degeneration in the fundus corresponds to the region left free after the lesions of area 19 in Cats 12 and 79 (Figs. 15 and 16) and is probably a separate field, but a continuation of the lateral suprasylvian area cannot be entirely ruled out.

There is a band of moderately heavy degeneration extending along the banks of the lateral sulcus and downwards across the upper part of the posterior suprasylvian gyrus to the splenial sulcus on the medial surface. It is obviously in area 19 and seems to fill most of its medio-lateral extent, but the degeneration is heaviest laterally. There is a second band of less dense degeneration running along most of the length of area 18 but concentrated near the 18–19 boundary. Further moderate degeneration is present in the dorsal bank of the splenial sulcus throughout most of its length. Adjacent Nissl sections indicate that this definitely occupies area 17 but, in the rostral half of the sulcus, it extends medially beyond the boundary of area 17 and as far as the fundus. It is complementary to the area in the fundus left free of degeneration after the lesion of area 7 in Cat 49 (Fig. 14). A few fragments are present on other parts of area 17 on the medial surface, especially caudally; near the representation of the area centralis on the dorsal surface, there is a small focus of quite dense terminal degeneration at the 17–18 boundary.

The distribution of degeneration in Cat 16 is similar though less and is more obviously concentrated in lateral parts of areas 18 and 19 and in medial parts of area 17 (including the adjacent small part of area 19 in the rostral half of the splenial sulcus). All these parts contain the representations of the periphery of the retina. In both brains, the concentration of degenerating fragments in areas 17, 18 and 19 is substantially less than in the lateral suprasylvian area after lesions of the other three. The frontal lobes of both brains contain terminal degeneration: this is in area 6aβ and is concentrated at the medial end of the cruciate sulcus, but some fragments are also present at the rostral end of the presylvian sulcus.

Area 20 (Cats 10, 68 and 70). In these experiments, as far as can be ascertained, the area of damage is confined within area 20 (Fig. 18). The ensuing terminal

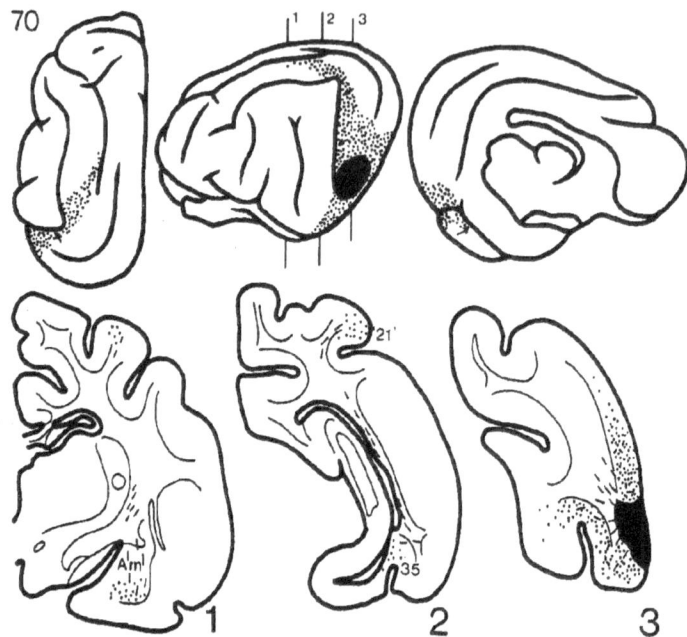

Fig. 18. An experiment in which a lesion of area 20 causes terminal degeneration throughout most of the posterior suprasylvian gyrus and extending rostrally along the lateral boundary of area 19 (in "area 21"). Additional degeneration extends inferiorly into the peri-rhinal area (35) and degenerating fibres distribute terminal fragments to the basolateral group of amygdaloid nuclei (*Am*, section 1)

degeneration fills area 20: caudally it reaches to the margin of area 19 in the caudal end of the splenial sulcus; rostrally, it extends for a short distance into the lower part of the posterior suprasylvian sulcus and, dorsally, it reaches upwards to fill that part of the posterior suprasylvian gyrus not occupied by area 19. This degeneration extends for a short distance into the caudal aspect of the medial bank of the middle suprasylvian sulcus and continues forwards into the middle suprasylvian gyrus along the lateral border of area 19. Ventral to the lesion, degeneration extends through the lateral bank of the rhinal sulcus to reach area 35 in the fundus. This degeneration is probably a little caudal to, but overlaps that seen in area 35 after the lesion of area 7 in Cat 49 (Fig. 16).

It is noteworthy that in all these brains with lesions of area 20, there is quite dense terminal degeneration in the basolateral group of amygdaloid nuclei (Fig. 32).

The Dorsal Part of the Posterior Suprasylvian Gyrus (Cats 46 and 71). The area of cortex situated at the upper part of the posterior suprasylvian gyrus and extending rostrally as a narrow strip between areas 7 and 19 was damaged in two experiments (Fig. 19). In these brains there are narrow strips of damage mainly along the caudal bank of the posterior suprasylvian sulcus in its dorsal few mm. Each of these lesions causes terminal degeneration in the upper half of the posterior

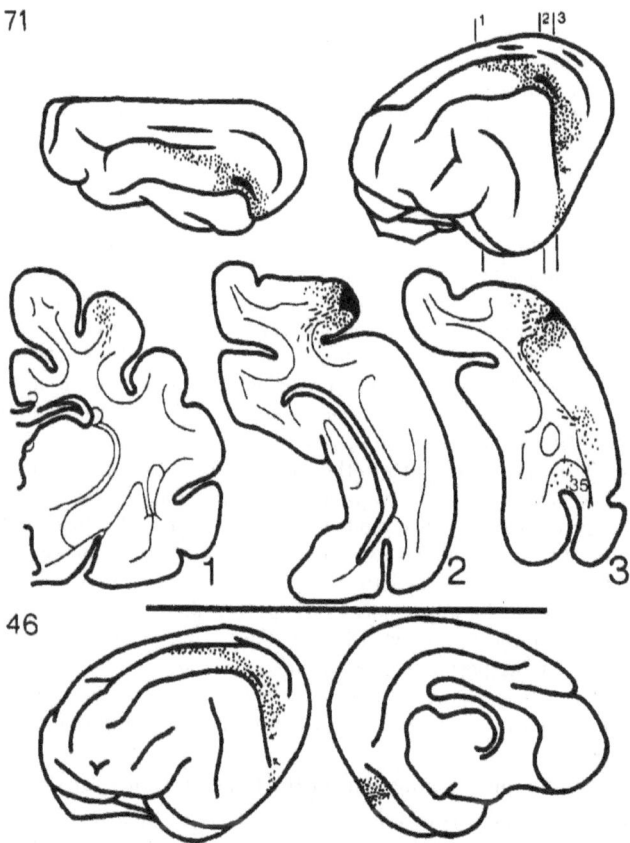

Fig. 19. Two experiments with small lesions of the unnamed area ("21") at the dorsal end of the posterior suprasylvian gyrus. Terminal degeneration extends forwards along the lateral margin of area 19 and downwards through the fundus of the posterior suprasylvian sulcus to the peri-rhinal cortex. The sections are from Cat 71 only

suprasylvian gyrus, in a small area bounded by area 19 dorsally and posteriorly, area 20 ventrally, and the posterior suprasylvian sulcus anteriorly. It encroaches slightly on the banks of the middle and posterior suprasylvian sulci close to their junction, in a region just dorsal and posterior to that occupied by the caudal extremity of the lateral suprasylvian area. It then continues rostrally along the lateral boundary of area 19 and, becoming progressively narrower, it disappears near the middle of the lateral sulcus. In both brains, there is an additional focus of fine, but quite dense terminal degeneration occupying the lower half of the fundus of the posterior suprasylvian sulcus and it appears to be separate from the degeneration in the area damaged. It does not extend caudally enough to affect area 20 but it extends to the rhinal sulcus over a small area immediately ventral to

Ep. It is probable that this degeneration occupies the same region as that seen in the posterior suprasylvian sulcus following lesions of field Ep and of the lateral suprasylvian area. In both brains, a few scattered degenerating fragments are also present in area 6 of the frontal cortex, chiefly in the lateral bank of the presylvian sulcus close to its rostral end.

Comment

These experiments offer confirmatory evidence for the individuality of the fields defined in earlier sections of the results. The following pattern of cortico-cortical connexions has emerged: area 5, which is the part of the suprasylvian gyrus directly connected to the primary somatic sensory cortex, sends fibres to area 7 locally and to a portion of area 6 in the frontal lobe. Area 7 then projects to the cingulate cortex, to the peri-rhinal cortex, and to the whole of area 6. Area 7 also receives fibres from the suprasylvian fringe, to which the auditory fields, AI, AII and Ep, project. The visually associated areas of the suprasylvian gyrus, i.e. area 19 and the lateral suprasylvian area, are reciprocally connected in an organized fashion corresponding to the retinal representation, with one another and with areas 17 and 18. Area 19 projects to area 20 at the lower part of the suprasylvian gyrus. This, in turn, sends fibres to an area in the dorsal half of the posterior suprasylvian gyrus and extending into the middle suprasylvian gyrus along the lateral boundary of area 19. Both of these areas have small projections to area 6; the area in the upper part of the gyrus, like the lateral suprasylvian area and Ep, has a projection to what is probably a separate area in the fundus of the ventral part of the posterior suprasylvian sulcus and extending to the peri-rhinal cortex ventral to Ep. Area 20 also sends fibres into the peri-rhinal cortex and has a projection to the basolateral group of amygdaloid nuclei.

Commissural Connexions of the Suprasylvian Gyrus

In the brains which have just been described, the individual areas of the middle and posterior suprasylvian gyri also exhibit characteristic patterns of commissural connexions.

In the brain in which *area 5* was damaged (Cat 1), terminal degeneration in the opposite hemisphere is confined to an almost symmetrical area (Fig. 20). A few degenerating fibres and terminals encroach on the caudal bank of the ansate sulcus and on the rostral aspect of the lateral gyrus, but these are still within area 5.

The lesion in *area 7* in Cat 49 caused suprisingly little degeneration in the contralateral hemisphere and this is restricted to the junction of areas 5 and 7 (Fig. 20). The remainder of the middle suprasylvian gyrus is free of fragments. This was confirmed in Cats 8 and 75 in which very large lesions destroyed most of the middle suprasylvian gyrus from area 5 rostrally to the postlateral sulcus caudally, and including large parts of area 19 and the lateral suprasylvian area. In the brain with the larger lesion (Cat 75), the upper half of the posterior suprasylvian gyrus has also been ablated. The distribution of degenerating axons in the contralateral cortex is virtually identical in the two cases (Fig. 20). A band of terminal degeneration conforming to area 5 spans the rostral part of the middle suprasylvian gyrus and from this, two streams of intense terminal degeneration extend caudally along the medial and lateral margins of the middle suprasylvian

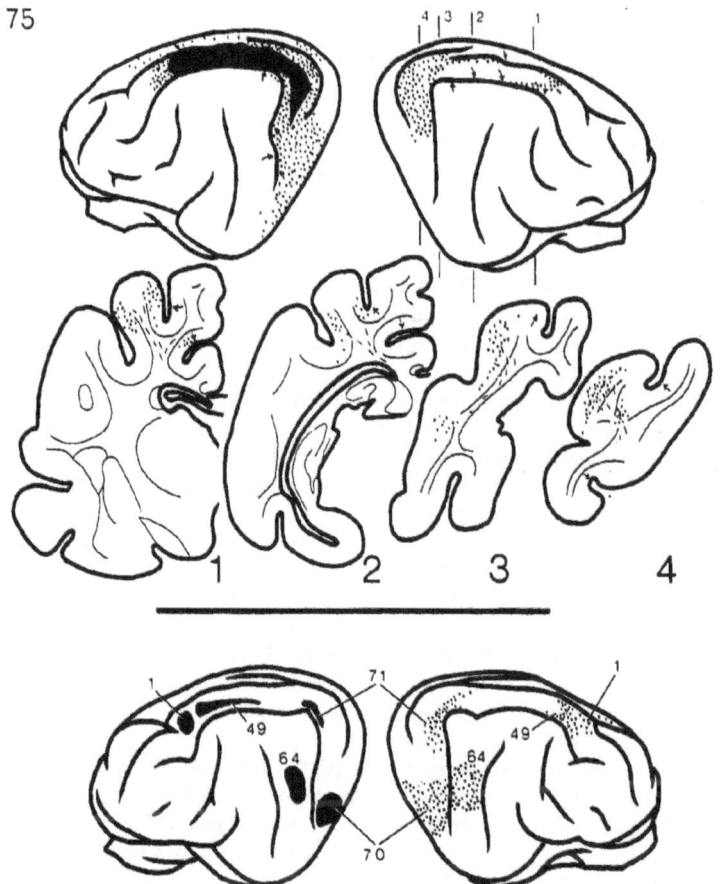

Fig. 20. Upper: the distribution of commissural fibres in an experiment in which large portions of the middle and posterior suprasylvian gyri were destroyed. Note the sparing of most of area 7 on the opposite side and the small focus of degeneration in the part of area 19 situated in the rostral part of the splenial sulcus (section 1). Lower: the distribution of degeneration in the contralateral cortex following lesions of certain parts of the suprasylvian gyrus. In most cases, the commissural degeneration fills an area of cortex which is approximately symmetrical to that destroyed by the lesion. However, a lesion of area 7 (Cat 49) causes degeneration only in the most rostral part of the opposite area 7

gyrus. One of these lies within area 19 although the part adjacent to area 18 is free of degeneration; the other occupies the medial bank of the middle suprasylvian sulcus in a region conforming to the lateral suprasylvian area, no part of which is free of degeneration. The two bands expand and meet in the caudal part of the middle suprasylvian gyrus and the fragments extend ventrally to fill most of the posterior suprasylvian gyrus with degeneration, particularly in Cat 75. In both brains, the greater part, if not all, of area 7 is free of degeneration.

The large lesion of *areas 17, 18 and 19* (Cat 12, see Fig. 16) causes commissural degeneration along the common boundary of areas 17 and 18, in the lateral half of area 19 and throughout the whole of the lateral suprasylvian area. It is interesting to note how the degeneration in the opposite area 19 of this brain (and also in Cats 8 and 75) almost encircles area 17, spreading into the rostral half and the caudal end of the splenial sulcus. In these parts of the sulcus, this degeneration in area 19 continues along the fundus adjacent to the boundary of area 17. As there is no degeneration in the adjoining area 17 of any of these brains, the small strip of terminal degeneration stands out very clearly. With the exception of the extreme caudal end, there is no degeneration near the medial boundary of area 17 in the caudal half of the sulcus.

After the small lesion confined to the caudal part of *area 19* in Cat 78 (see Fig. 11), degenerating commissural fibres and their terminals are found in a small focus in a symmetrical part of area 19 and in the fundus of the opposite middle suprasylvian sulcus, close to what has been identified as the caudal end of the lateral suprasylvian area.

The two lesions of the *lateral suprasylvian area* (Cats 16 and 32, see Fig. 17) cause degeneration only in the opposite lateral suprasylvian area. That in Cat 16 (the smaller lesion affecting the representation of the periphery of the retina), occupies mainly the outer part of the medial bank of the middle suprasylvian sulcus but it extends for the full length of the lateral suprasylvian area. In the brain with the larger lesion (Cat 32), the whole of the opposite lateral suprasylvian area is filled with fragments, although the intensity is rather less at the rostral and caudal ends of the medial bank.

Following the three lesions of *area 20* (Cats 10, 68 and 70, see Fig. 12) and the two of the area at the upper end of the posterior suprasylvian gyrus (Cats 46 and 71, see Figs. 12 and 18), commissural degeneration is confined to the homotopical area and fills a region which in size and position is virtually a mirror image of that destroyed by the lesion (Fig. 20).

Comment

Areas 5, 20 and the unnamed area at the upper end of the posterior suprasylvian gyrus have commissural connexions only with their counterparts in the opposite cortex. Area 7 either has no commissural connexions, or these are restricted to its extreme rostral end. Area 19, like areas 17 and 18, has commissural connexions only between those portions containing the representation of the parts of the retina adjoining the vertical meridian. These connexions furnish additional evidence for an extension of area 19 onto the medial surface of the brain but only in the rostral half and the extreme caudal end of the splenial sulcus. Area 19 also sends commissural fibres to the opposite lateral suprasylvian area but the latter has such connexions only with its counterpart. No part of the lateral suprasylvian area fails to receive commissural fibres but they may be less densely distributed to its extremities. Most of these results are in accord with those previously reported by Ebner and Myers (1965), Hubel and Wiesel (1965), Garey et al. (1968) and Wilson (1968).

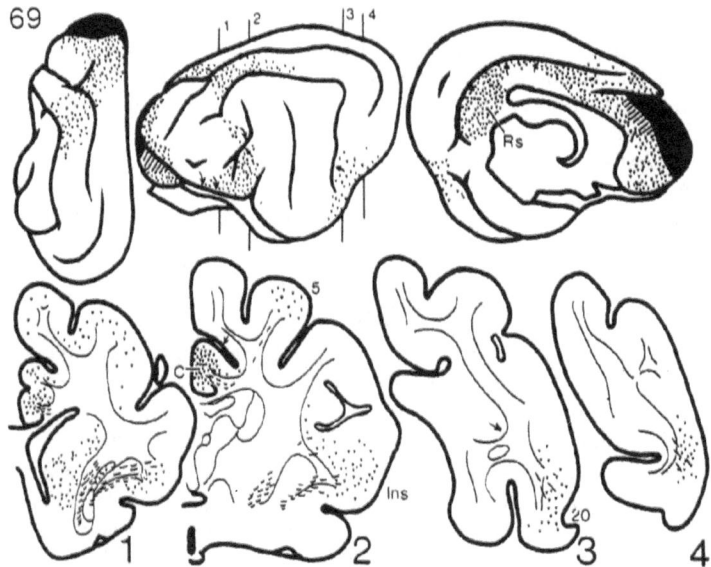

Fig. 21. A large lesion of the frontal lobe (the hatched part is subcortical only) which causes degeneration in areas 5 and 7 at the rostral end of the middle suprasylvian gyrus and in area 20 of the posterior suprasylvian gyrus. Additional degeneration affects the insular area, the rostral part of the cingulate area and the whole retrosplenial area. The small foci of degeneration in the hindlimb areas of SI and SII result from damage of the hindlimb part of the motor cortex

Connexions of the Frontal Cortex

Since many of the areas in the suprasylvian gyrus have projections to the frontal lobe, it is of interest to determine to what extent these are reciprocated by fibres returning from the frontal cortex.

Cat 69. A large lesion was made by suction in the frontal lobe (Fig. 21). The whole gyrus proreus has been ablated and the rostral half of the ventral bank of the cruciate sulcus removed. The medial surface of the remaining portion of the frontal lobe and the medial bank of the presylvian sulcus are undercut by an extension of the lesion into the white matter. The whole orbito-frontal cortex has been removed, together with most of area 6 and there is involvement of the anterior limbic area. A small amount of damage to the hindlimb area of the motor cortex is reflected in foci of axonal degeneration in the hindlimb subdivisions of SI and of SII. Degenerating axons can be traced through the external capsule and claustrum to the insular cortex, where they distribute moderately heavy terminal degeneration. Others pass through the equivalent of the cingulum to two parts of the cingulate gyrus. One of these conforms almost exactly to the retrosplenial area of Rose and Woolsey (1948b). The degeneration in it commences as a narrow band abutting on the medial boundary of area 17 in the middle part of the splenial sulcus and the degeneration continues in contact with area 17 as far as the caudal end of the sulcus. The other fills the anterior limbic area but also invades the rostral half of the "cingulate area" of Rose and Woolsey in the middle part of the cingulate gyrus; it continues caudally along the ventral bank of the splenial sulcus almost as far as the commencement of the retrosplenial area.

The rostral ends of the splenial, lateral and middle suprasylvian gyri contain heavy degeneration in a region conforming to area 5 with possible extension into the rostral part of area 7. Sparse terminal degeneration is also present in area 20 and in the fundus of the posterior suprasylvian sulcus.

IV. Discussion

The results raise a number of significant points which, although inter-related, will be discussed separately for the sake of clarity.

Functional Localization in the Suprasylvian Gyrus

Certain aspects of the results are relevant to physiological studies which have dealt with functional localization in the suprasylvian gyrus. The relation of area 5 to the third somatic sensory area of Darian-Smith et al. (1966) has been considered in detail elsewhere (Jones and Powell, 1968a, 1969a) and it has been proposed that it is the "supplementary sensory area" observed in human patients and in the squirrel monkey (Penfield and Jasper, 1954; Blomquist and Lorenzini, 1965). Because its thalamic input is from the lateralis posterior nucleus, and not from the ventrobasal complex, area 5 should be considered in a different light from SI and SII. Furthermore, unlike SI and SII which are reciprocally connected, area 5 receives fibres from only one of them (SI) and does not return fibres to either of them.

Area 7, in its position, corresponds quite closely to Woolsey's (1961) area of auditory "association cortex" (Fig. 1), in which responses are obtained, after long latency, to auditory stimulation. That it is related to the auditory system is shown by the fact that it receives fibres from the suprasylvian fringe to which three of the primary auditory fields distribute fibres. In an earlier study (Diamond et al., 1968a), it was considered on the basis of one experiment that Ep probably also sent fibres to the middle suprasylvian gyrus, but it was not appreciated at the time just how low the suprasylvian fringe extended in the posterior ectosylvian gyrus. A part of the latter was almost certainly involved in the single experiment of Diamond et al. since a projection from Ep to the suprasylvian gyrus has not been confirmed in the present study.

Although areas 5 and 7 do not receive fibres from the somatic sensory and auditory relay nuclei of the thalamus it is possible that somatic sensory and auditory information may reach them by routes other than the cortico-cortical. Each receives fibres from the lateralis posterior nucleus which is the recipient of fibres from the superior colliculus, to which the ascending somatic and auditory pathways distribute fibres (Woollard and Harpman, 1940; Nauta and Kuypers, 1958; Mehler, 1969).

Area 19 and the lateral suprasylvian area are obviously parts of the cortical visual system (Hubel and Wiesel, 1965, 1969) and have been extensively studied with electrophysiological techniques. The present results confirm other studies in showing that areas 17, 18, 19 and the lateral suprasylvian area are reciprocally connected by cortico-cortical fibres (Hubel and Wiesel, 1965; Garey et al., 1968; Wilson, 1968; Heath and Jones, 1970). Although the axonal degeneration occurring in areas 17, 18 and 19 after a lesion of the lateral suprasylvian area is appreciably less than in the latter after a lesion of the other three, it is consistent and follows the representational pattern. The distribution of degeneration in relation to the representation pattern offers support for the physiological observations of Hubel and Wiesel (1969) on the representation in the lateral suprasylvian area. They found that the periphery of the visual field was represented in the more superficial part of the medial bank of the middle suprasylvian sulcus and the vertical meridian nearer the fundus. The present experiments show that a lesion of the more superficial part (Cat 16, Fig. 17) causes degeneration in the parts of areas 17, 18 and 19 representing the periphery and that as deeper parts of the lateral suprasylvian area are affected (Cat 32, Fig. 17), so the degeneration moves more towards the representation of the vertical meridian.

Unlike the other three visual areas in which the representations of the periphery of the visual field are not commissurally connected (Choudhury, Whitteridge and Wilson, 1965; Berlucchi, Gazzaniga and Rizzolatti, 1967; Garey et al., 1968; Hubel and Wiesel, 1967; Wilson, 1968), all parts of the two lateral suprasylvian areas are connected across the midline by such fibres. However, the intensity of commissural degeneration in one lateral suprasylvian area after a lesion of its counterpart is less at its rostral and caudal ends. It is possible, therefore, that if a good deal of the peripheral representation is crowded into the ends, as in areas 17, 18 and 19 (Hubel and Wiesel, 1965), then the peripheral representation may receive fewer commissural fibres.

The lateral suprasylvian area appears to be restricted to the rostro-caudal extent of the middle suprasylvian sulcus (Fig. 22), crossing from its medial to its lateral bank at the caudal end of the sulcus. In the experiments with damage of the lateral suprasylvian area, degeneration in the undamaged portions of the area reached downwards into the fundus of the posterior suprasylvian sulcus, so that the possibility exists that the lateral suprasylvian area could, in fact, extend this far also. The observations of Hubel and Wiesel (1969) that in the part of the lateral suprasylvian area which they studied (approximately in the middle of the middle suprasylvian sulcus), most neurons were related to parts of the retina lying below the horizontal meridian, might be taken as evidence for this; by comparison with the other visual areas, the representation of the superior half of the retina should be posteriorly situated and equally large as that of the inferior half. Against this, however, are the facts that lesions involving the representation of the superior retina in areas 17 and 18 or 19 did not cause degeneration of corticocortical fibres in the lateral suprasylvian area to spread more caudally than the junction of the middle and posterior suprasylvian sulci. Conversely, lesions of the part of the lateral suprasylvian area in the middle suprasylvian sulcus did cause degeneration in caudal parts of areas 17, 18 and 19 in which the superior retina is represented. Finally, these lesions of the lateral suprasylvian area caused degeneration only in the middle suprasylvian sulcus of the opposite side. Therefore, with the reservations expressed above, it seems probable that the area in the fundus of

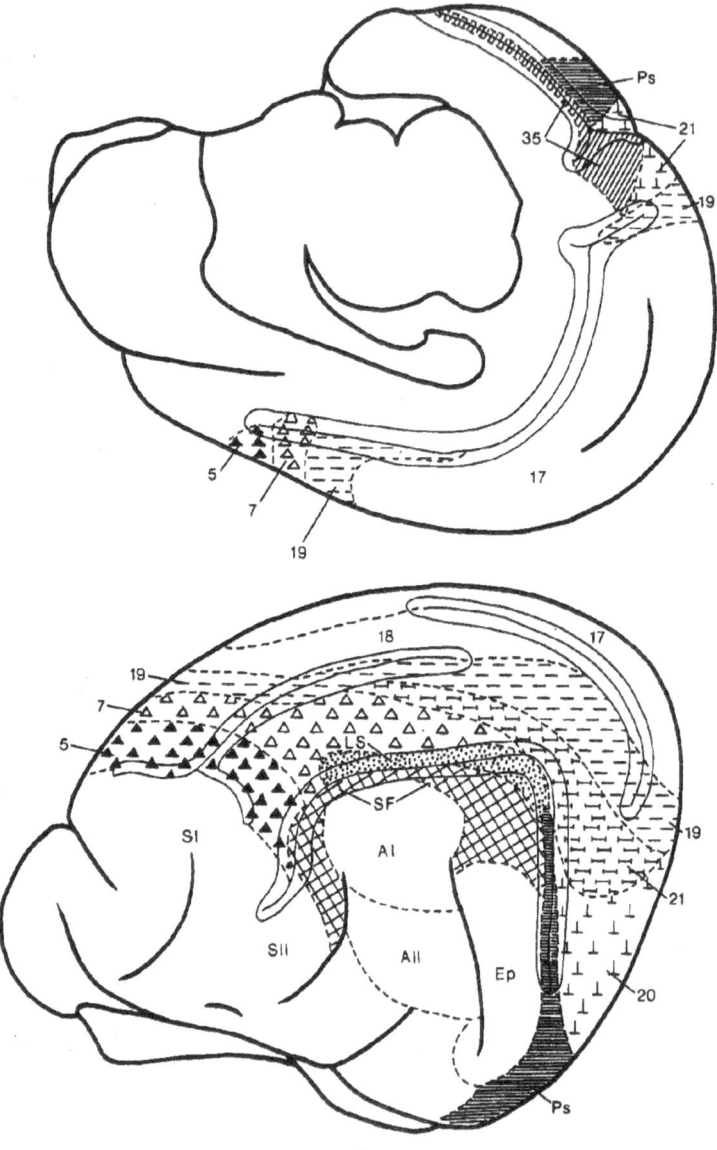

Fig. 22. A schematic diagram showing the distribution and relative dispositions of the cortical fields in the suprasylvian gyrus, as defined on the basis of their connexions in the present study. The adjacent somatic, auditory and visual fields are also indicated following various authors (see text). This figure should be compared with the architectonic maps given in Fig. 1

the posterior suprasylvian sulcus, though receiving fibres from the lateral supra-sylvian area, is a separate field from the latter.

The limits of area 19 have been defined on the basis of cortico-cortical, thalamo-cortical and commissural connexions (Fig. 22). On this basis, it appears that area 19 forms a C-shaped field almost encircling area 17. On the medial surface of the hemisphere, it separates area 17 from the limbic cortex in the rostral half and at the extreme caudal end of the splenial sulcus, but elsewhere in the splenial sulcus, area 17 abuts directly on the cingulate or retrosplenial cortex.

Another small area responsive to visual stimuli has been described at the junction of the anterior and middle suprasylvian sulci by Landgren and Silf-venius (1969). This lies mainly in the medial bank of the sulcus but overlaps an auditory projection area in the lateral bank, and vestibular and somatic sensory projection areas situated a little more anteriorly in the sulcus (Landgren, Silf-venius and Wolsk, 1967). Landgren and his colleagues consider that this region, therefore, plays "a role in the animal's orientation against [sic] sound stimuli" and "the orientation of the eyes towards suddenly occurring sounds". The present results, taken in conjunction with those of Heath and Jones (1971) who demon-strated the projection of the suprageniculate and magnocellular medial genicu-culate nuclei to the cortex, suggest that several distinct areas come into apposition in this small region at the junction of the two parts of the suprasylvian sulcus (Fig. 22). These include extensions of areas 5 and 7, and the vestibular projection area (Walzl and Mountcastle, 1949; Mickle and Ades, 1952); immediately rostral to these the representations of the occipital region in SI and of the trigeminal nerve in SII come together (Woolsey, 1958); caudally, they abut on the supra-sylvian fringe and the lateral suprasylvian area. Therefore, it is doubtful whether the region described by Landgren and his co-workers should be considered as an independent entity with a specific function.

The other areas of the middle and posterior suprasylvian gyri as defined by their connexions—areas 7, 20 and the area intercalated between these and area 19—have not been defined electrophysiologically. It may be noted, however, that area 20 and the unnamed intercalated area just mentioned, represent the second and third steps in an outward cortico-cortical progression from the visual areas. Therefore, it would be interesting to study them with microelectrodes to determine whether the increasing complexity of stimuli required to fire neurons in passing from area 17, through area 18 to area 19 (Hubel and Wiesel, 1965), is continued. Since the unnamed area receives fibres from area 20 it bears the same relationship to the visual areas as does area 21 of the monkey (Jones and Powell, 1970a) and it seems not unreasonable to regard it as the homologue of area 21 (Fig. 22).

Relation to Architectonic Maps

Throughout the present experiments, we have attempted to relate the bound-aries of the fields defined on a connexional basis to architectonic boundaries visible in the same brain. However, in experimental material and particularly in those areas whose boundaries do not show a sharp architectonic change (eg. the lateral boundary of area 19), this has not always been possible. In this regard, it is inter-esting to relate the findings based on connexions (Fig. 22) to those of workers who

have subdivided the suprasylvian gyrus on strictly morphological grounds
(Fig. 1). In general, where in our experience a field has clear-cut boundaries, the
parcellations of two or more other workers are usually in accord with one another,
and their field is usually coincident with one based on connexions alone. Area 5
is a good example of this. The large cells of layer V make it distinct even in Nauta-
stained sections; Gurewitsch and Chatschaturian (1928), Hassler and Muhs-
Clement (1964) and Sanides and Hoffmann (1969) (who call it "a parietal integration belt") agree quite closely on its boundaries, and its distinctive cortical and
thalamic connexions respect these boundaries. On the other hand, where a field
has one or more indistinct boundaries, students of architectonics will generally
disagree as to the extent of the field, and the field as defined by connexions may
not conform to any of their delimitations. Areas 7 and 19 are cases in point: the
rostral boundary of the one and the medial boundary of the other are quite sharp
and there is little disagreement about these. However, the medial boundary of
area 7 and the lateral boundary of area 19 are indistinct and there is considerable
disagreement as to the positions of the boundaries. Significantly, the boundaries
of these areas as defined by connexions, do not conform to any of the published
maps. For example, in the present results, the lateral boundary of area 19
approximately follows that defined by Otsuka and Hassler (1962) in its rostral
half but, towards the caudal end of the middle suprasylvian gyrus, it moves
further laterally to lie closer to that defined for the peristriate belt by Sanides
and Hoffmann (1969). Then instead of continuing downwards into the posterior
suprasylvian gyrus as shown by the latter workers, it again follows the line drawn
by Otsuka and Hassler across the caudal surface of the hemisphere. On the medial
aspect of the brain, Otsuka and Hassler claim that a strip of area 19 lies in contiguity with the medial boundary of area 17 throughout the whole rostro-caudal
extent of the splenial sulcus; Sanides and Hoffmann are adamant that this is
not area 19 but a part of the limbic cortex. The present results suggest that the
true situation lies somewhere between these two extremes, for area 19 as defined
by connexions, does lie adjacent to area 17 but only in the rostral half and at the
extreme caudal end of the splenial sulcus. In the rest of the sulcus, narrow extensions of the cingulate and retrosplenial areas lie adjacent to area 17. Therefore,
the extent of area 19 as based on architectonic criteria alone, will depend upon
how much one's decision is governed by the appearances present in sections
through the rostral or caudal halves of the splenial sulcus. The present results
meet the desideratum of Woolsey (1947) that area 17 should be, over some of its
extent, in contiguity with limbic cortex.

The lack of agreement between architectonic maps and the delimitation of
fields on the basis of connexions is even more striking in the posterior suprasylvian
gyrus. Sanides and Hoffmann (1969) virtually fill the gyrus with their equivalent
of area 19, except for its ventral portion which they regard as "paralimbic cortex"
and its rostral part which they regard as a continuation of the "suprasylvian
sulcus belt". Otsuka and Hassler (1962) do not take area 19 into the posterior
suprasylvian gyrus, except along the lateral bank of the postlateral sulcus.
Gurewitsch and Chatschaturian (1928) take area 18 across the dorsal aspect of the
gyrus and fill the rest with parts of areas 21, 20 and 36, in succession from dorsal
to ventral. On a connexional basis, area 19 occupies only the upper part of the

gyrus, area 18 and the lateral suprasylvian area do not extend into it, and there are distinct fields in the dorsal and ventral aspects of the gyrus and probably in the fundus of the posterior suprasylvian sulcus. The disagreement between architectonic maps in the posterior suprasylvian gyrus doubtless reflects the difficulty of drawing boundary lines across a region of cortex which is not only fairly uniform in structure but which, in being near the caudal pole, rapidly changes its orientation in all the standard planes of section.

Significance of Architectonic Subdivisions

The present study, especially when taken in conjunction with one on the cortico-cortical connexions of the parieto-temporal region in the monkey (Jones, 1969; Jones and Powell, 1970a), lends added weight to current arguments in favour of the significance of cortical architectonics. Following the detailed and in the light of contemporary evidence, unreasonable parcellations of the Vogts (Vogt and Vogt, 1919), architectonic studies of the cortex fell into disrepute (see for example Lashley and Clark, 1946; Bailey and Bonin, 1951). Recently, however, there has been a revival of interest in such studies for it has become obvious that in the primary sensory areas at least, architectural differences do, indeed, betoken differences in the physiological properties of their constituent neurons (Powell and Mountcastle, 1959; Hubel and Wiesel, 1965). The evidence that three diverse sets of connexions—associational, commissural and thalamo-cortical—respect the boundaries of individual architectonic fields in the primary sensory areas, argues further in favour of these fields being valid entities (eg. Rose and Woolsey, 1948a, b, 1949a, b, 1958; Hubel and Wiesel, 1965; Jones and Powell, 1968a, b, 1969a, b, c, 1970a, b; Diamond et al., 1968a, b, 1969). Therefore, provided they are viewed in conjunction with their connexions and with the properties of their contained neurons, architectonic areas must be of functional significance; differences in either one of structure, connexions or response properties could, then, indicate differences in function. On this basis, some areas although having a transitional structure would become highly specific fields if their connexions or the response properties of their neurons were to be different from those of adjoining fields. One case in point is that of areas 21 and 20 of the monkey temporal lobe: although considered separate fields by Brodmann (1909), they were classed as one by Bonin and Bailey (1947) because of similarities in structure. Yet their connexions are different (Jones and Powell, 1970a) and experimental psychological studies have been able to distinguish different effects on visual discriminations following lesions of the anterior (area 21) and posterior (area 20) parts of the infero-temporal region (Weiskrantz, 1968). This example is particularly relevant to the present study because areas 20 and 21 are the second and third steps in a chain of cortico-cortical connexions passing outwards from the visual areas, and from the present study, they appear to have their counterparts in the cat.

In considering the significance of cortical architectonics, it must be remembered that all areas of the cortex have an overall similarity in structure and although differences in structure and connexions must reflect differences in function, the converse is also true (Le Gros Clark, 1952). The similarity in structure of the large tracts of homotypical cortex of the frontal, temporal and parietal lobes obviously impressed such authors as Bailey and Bonin (1951) far more than the differences had impressed Brodmann and his followers; Bailey and Bonin were, therefore, reluctant to subdivide the cortex as far as had the latter. However, the two views are not necessarily irreconcilable. Within these regions in the primate and to a considerable extent even in the cat, there are clearly individual projection areas of the visual, auditory and somatic sensory cortex, but the basic similarity in the organization of the pathways proceeding outwards from these primary areas (Jones and Powell, 1970a) may reflect a further similarity in the manner in which information is processed in each pathway. On these grounds, the "association" areas in each pathway may be expected to display a similar structure.

Obviously, the cortico-cortical is probably not the only connexion which may impose a structural design upon the subdivisions of the cortex. The commissural and thalamo-cortical are almost certainly also involved. Thus, it would be theoretically possible to make different subdivisions of the cortex on the basis of each of the three types of connexion. Up to the present, however, all the evidence indicates that the boundaries of a field determined by one set of connexions generally coincide with those delimited by the others. Possible exceptions may occur, particularly in the somatic sensory and visual areas where some parts—the representations respectively of the distal aspects of the limbs and of the periphery of the visual field—lack commissural connexions. Sanides and Hoffmann (1969) and Sanides and Krishnamurti (1967) in the somatic sensory areas of the cat and slow loris, and Kaas, Hall and Diamond (1970) in the visual cortex of the hedgehog, claim to be able to distinguish architectonic differences between these and other parts of the representation.

Thalamic Connexions of the Suprasylvian Gyrus

The present results on the thalamic connexions of the suprasylvian gyrus confirm and extend what has been broadly known for some time, chiefly from studies with the cell degeneration technique (Waller and Barris, 1937). It is obvious that the middle and posterior suprasylvian gyri are related to the whole complex of nuclei comprising the lateralis dorsalis, lateralis posterior and posterior nuclei, and the pulvinar. The problem of obtaining uncomplicated lesions in this part of the thalamus makes a comprehensive study of the thalamo-cortical connexions by the method of anterograde degeneration a difficult one. However, by comparing several experiments with lesions of the thalamus with one another, and with the results of experiments on the reciprocal, cortico-thalamic pathway, it has been possible to arrive at certain general conclusions concerning the thalamic relationships of the suprasylvian gyrus.

Probably the thalamic connexions of the four visual areas are of the greatest topical interest, for these have been repeatedly studied with both the anterograde axonal and the retrograde cellular degeneration techniques. Although there is some disagreement regarding the finer details of the projection, most workers have regarded the dorsal lateral geniculate nucleus as projecting to all four areas (Garey and Powell, 1967; Wilson and Cragg, 1967; Glickstein et al., 1967; Niimi and Sprague, 1970). Recently, however, it has been suggested by Graybiel (1970) that the main source of afferents to area 19 and the lateral suprasylvian area is the

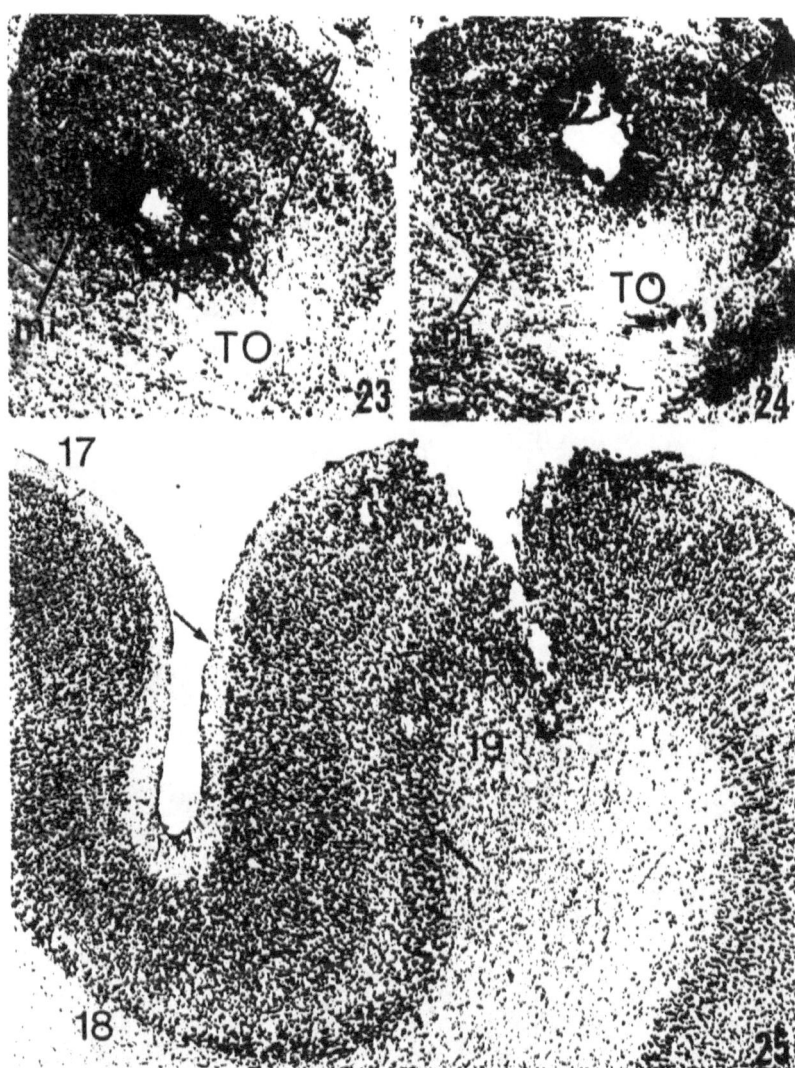

Figs. 23 and 24. The lesions of the lateral geniculate nuclei in Cats 40L (23) and 40R (24) (see also Figs. 3 and 4). The photomicrographs are taken from the levels of maximal extent of the lesions. The main laminae of the dorsal lateral geniculate nucleus are, in each case, indicated by arrows. The lesion in 40L (Fig. 23) affects primarily lamina B and the medial interlaminar nucleus (*mi*). That in 40R (Fig. 24) damages only the main laminae. TO: optic tract. Thionin stain, ×15

Fig. 25. A photomicrograph of the lesion of area 19 in Cat 78 (Fig. 15), at its level of maximal extent. The architectonic boundary between areas 18 and 19 is clearly visible and is indicated by the arrows. Thionin stain, ×15

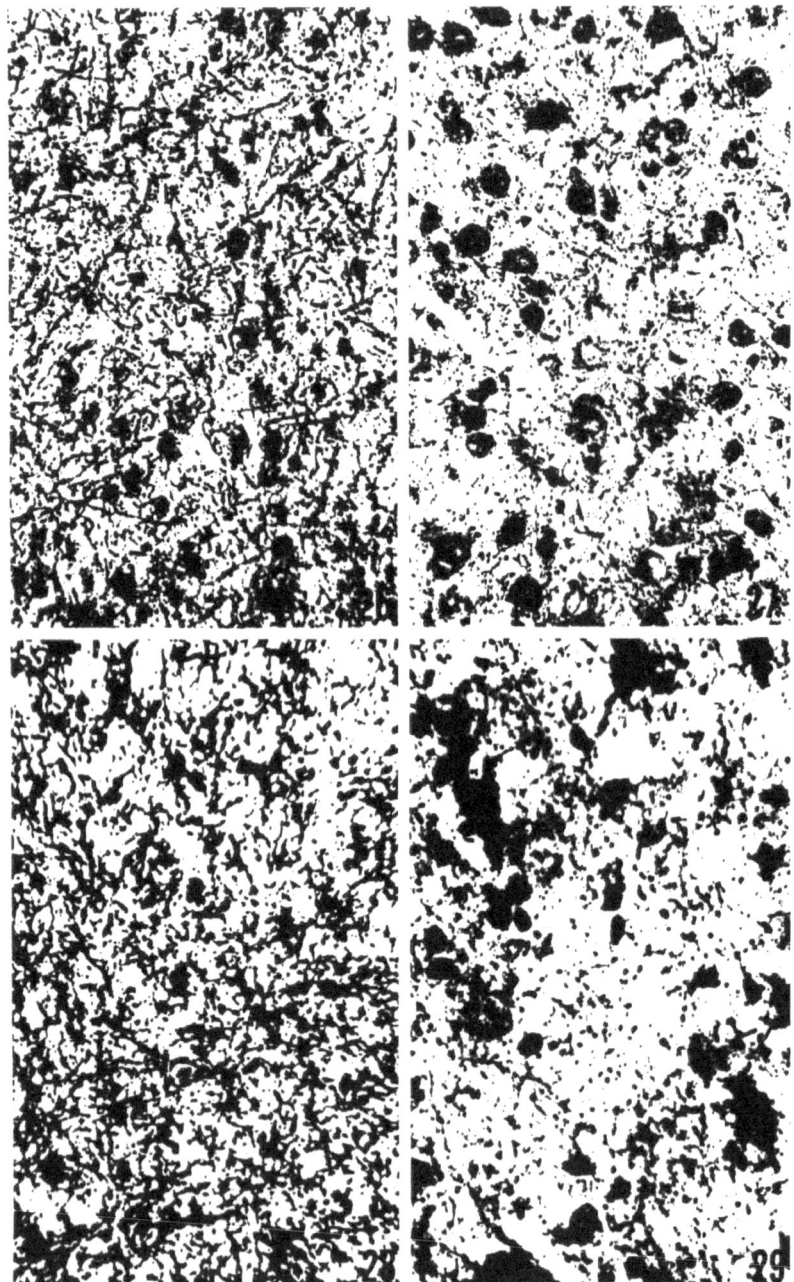

Figs. 26–29

lateralis posterior-pulvinar complex. Graybiel indicates that fibres passing to the cortex from the latter traverse the dorsal lateral geniculate nucleus. The present results are in accord with those of Graybiel and although it is not possible to rule out completely a small projection to area 19 and the lateral suprasylvian area from the main laminae or the medial interlaminar nucleus, it appears more likely that the main laminae, at least, are projecting only to areas 17 and 18. Area 19 and the lateral suprasylvian area undoubtedly receive their heaviest, if not their sole thalamic input from the lateral nuclear complex (see also Burrows and Hayhow, 1970).

Even if this is accepted, there remains several aspects of the organization of the thalamic connexions of the visual pathways which are puzzling. One of the more prominent concerns the fact that although in other systems there is a firm interlocking by reciprocal connexions of a principal thalamic nucleus and its cortical target, this arrangement does not appear to hold in the visual system. The lateralis posterior nucleus is clearly the principal nucleus projecting to the middle suprasylvian gyrus, including area 19 and the lateral suprasylvian area, and these return fibres to it. However, areas 17 and 18 which do not receive fibres from the lateralis posterior-posterior complex, also send cortico-thalamic fibres to the same part of the lateralis posterior (see also Guillery, 1967; Garey et al., 1968; Holländer, 1970). This must have the effect of making the lateralis posterior quite different from the sensory relay nuclei which receive cortico-thalamic fibres only from the area of the cortex to which they send thalamo-cortical axons (Jones and Powell, 1968b, 1970b; Diamond et al., 1969; present study). Possibly it indicates that a greater degree of visual and even of polysensory convergence has occurred in the superior colliculus which is the main source of afferents to the lateral nuclear complex (Altman, 1962; Altman and Carpenter, 1961; Jassik-Gerschenfeld, 1966): all ascending sensory pathways and most parts of the cortex project to the superior colliculus (Jassik-Gerschenfeld, 1966; Kuypers and Lawrence, 1967; Garey et al., 1968). Convergence at the level of both the superior colliculus and the lateralis posterior might have as great an effect in making the peripheral receptive fields of neurons in areas 19 and the lateral suprasylvian area more complex than those in areas 17 and 18 (Hubel and Wiesel, 1965, 1969), as cortico-cortical fibres converging on area 19 and the lateral suprasylvian area from the other two.

Although the lateral nuclear complex is relatively homogeneous in structure, it is clear from the present results that parts of it are related to specific areas of the cortex, albeit with a certain amount of overlap especially in the rostral part of the

Fig. 26. Coarse axonal and terminal degeneration in the lateral suprasylvian area following a large lesion of the caudal thalamus involving the n. lateralis posterior. Nauta and Gygax stain, × 400

Fig. 27. Fine axonal and terminal degeneration in area 20 of the same brain from which Fig. 26 was taken, and at the same magnification. Nauta and Gygax stain, × 400

Fig. 28. Intense, coarse axonal and terminal degeneration in the n. lateralis posterior following a lesion of area 19. Nauta and Gygax stain, × 650

Fig. 29. Sparse, fine axonal and terminal degeneration in the pulvinar following a lesion of the upper part of the posterior suprasylvian gyrus. Nauta and Gygax stain, × 650

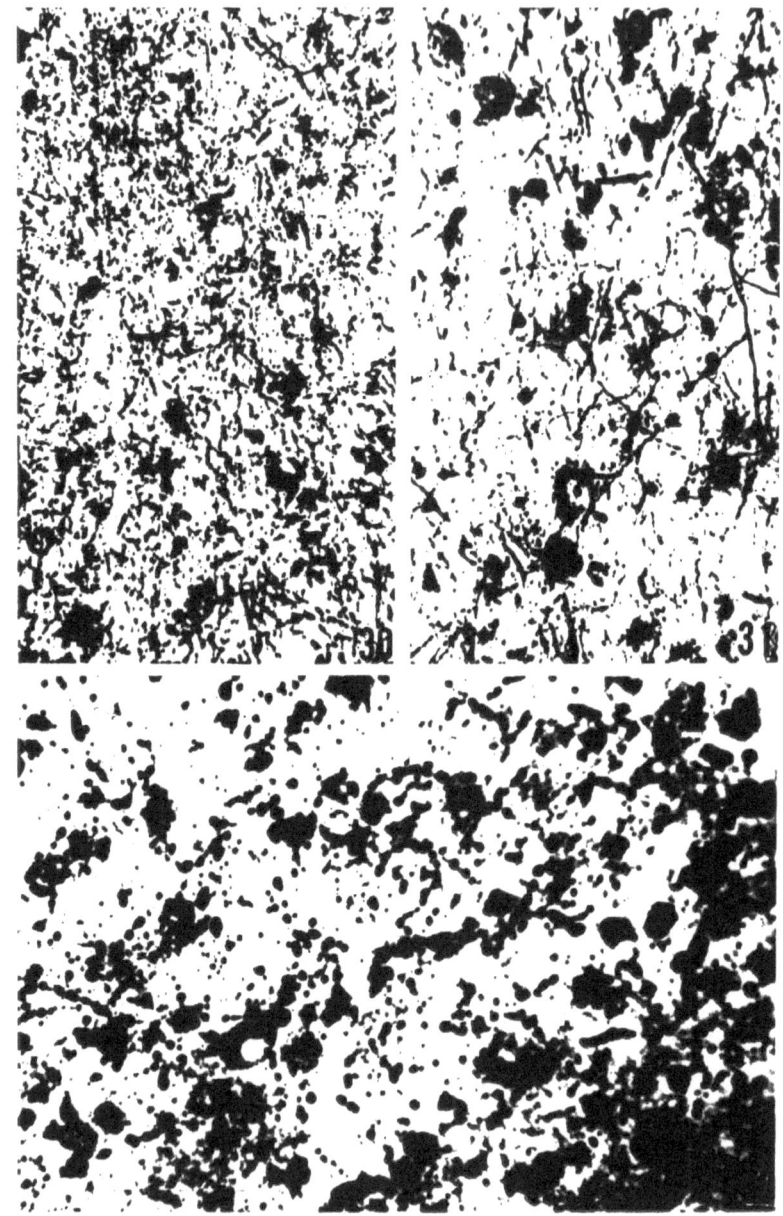

Fig. 30. Intense, coarse axonal and terminal degeneration in area 18 following a small lesion of area 19. Nauta and Gygax stain, ×500

Fig. 31. Sparse, fine axonal and terminal degeneration in area 20, photographed in the same section and at the same magnification as Fig. 30. Nauta and Gygax stain, ×500

Fig. 32. Terminal degeneration in the basolateral amygdala following a lesion of area 20. Fink and Heimer stain, ×1000

lateralis posterior nucleus. It would be interesting to know whether this overlap merely reflects the limitations of the present techniques or whether it is a reflection of a degree of inter-system convergence occurring in the superior colliculus (Jassik-Gerschenfeld, 1966) and then projected on to the lateralis posterior. If this were so, then the progressive cortico-cortical convergence of the sensory systems within the parts of the cortex related to the lateral nuclear complex (Jones and Powell, 1970a), could have its counterpart in the ascending subcortical pathways converging on the lateral nuclear complex *via* the superior colliculus. Hence, the ultimate area of cortico-cortical convergence between all sensory systems in the parieto-temporal region could also be the target of the part of the lateral nuclear complex or pulvinar showing complete convergence, *via* the superior colliculus, of all sensory systems. Since projections from the retina and from visually related areas of the cortex predominate in both the superior colliculus and the lateral nuclear-pulvinar complex, they could be significant in determining the role played by the former in visually guided behaviour (Schneider, 1969) and for the marked increase in size exhibited by the latter in animals such as the primates in whom visually guided behaviour is so dominant.

The cortical relationships of the pulvinar of the cat now seem established. From the results of experiments with lesions in the thalamus and in the cortex, it would appear that the ventral part of the pulvinar projects to area 20 and the remainder to the area in the upper part of the posterior suprasylvian gyrus which extends rostrally along the lateral margin of area 19. If there is a separate area in the fundus of the posterior suprasylvian sulcus, it too, probably receives fibres from the pulvinar. The distribution of the densest cortical degeneration following lesions made in the pulvinar by electrodes which traversed the suprasylvian gyrus, corpus callosum and medial parts of the thalamus (Clüver and Campos, 1970), is in accord with the present results.

It was noticeable in our experiments that nearly all the connexions of those areas more distantly removed from the primary sensory areas, but including area Ep (Diamond *et al.*, 1969), were composed of extremely fine fibres which distributed relatively sparse patterns of terminal degeneration (Figs. 26–31). This was particularly true of the cortico-thalamic connexions but was also evident in the thalamo-cortical, cortico-cortical and commissural. We do not know the significance of this and we are uncertain as to whether it necessarily implies that these areas, which would be construed as "association cortex", are phylogenetically older than the primary sensory areas (Bishop, 1959; Diamond and Hall, 1969).

Convergence in the Suprasylvian Gyrus

One of the main objects of the present study was to try to determine those areas of the suprasylvian gyrus in which cortico-cortical pathways emanating from the primary sensory areas might converge, as a possible guide towards understanding the polysensory areas of the anterior sigmoid, lateral and middle suprasylvian gyri. It should be stated at the outset that although the cortico-cortical pathways emanating from the primary sensory areas may ultimately converge, only one of the regions of convergence (area 6) even approximately coincides with one of the polysensory areas (the pre-cruciate area of the anterior sigmoid gyrus). Slightly different parts of area 6 receive cortico-cortical fibres from areas in the suprasylvian gyrus which are primarily related to the somatic, visual or auditory systems. The antero-medial end of the ventral bank of the cruciate sulcus (a part of area 6aβ of Hassler and Muhs-Clement, 1964) receives fibres from SI and SII (Jones and Powell, 1968a) and from the visual areas; the auditory fields project to most of area 6aβ (Diamond *et al.*, 1969). There is, thus, a good deal of overlap even in the frontal projections of the primary sensory areas. To this is added the projections of areas 5 and 7 which, together, fill the whole of area 6 including all three subdivisions of Hassler and Muhs-Clement. There is, therefore, an anatomical basis for equating area 6 with the pre-cruciate polysensory area. Similar conclusions have been drawn in the squirrel and rhesus monkeys (Bignall and Imbert, 1969; Jones and Powell, 1970a). This is not to say that cortico-cortical connexions are solely responsible for the multimodal convergence occurring in this or in any other polysensory area. Polysensory responses, although sometimes modified, usually survive ablation of the primary sensory cortex (Bignall, 1967, 1970; Rutledge and Shellenberger, 1968; Bignall and Imbert, 1969). However, convergence of cortico-cortical pathways related to several sensory systems may reflect similar convergence occurring at lower levels and projected on to the polysensory cortex.

Apart from area 6, in no other part of the cat brain do polysensory areas and regions of cortico-cortical convergence coincide. Yet in the three remaining polysensory areas there is clearly convergence upon many cells of somatic, auditory and visual impulses (see Thompson, 1967 for a review). It may be significant, however, that two of the polysensory areas—those at the rostral ends of the lateral and middle suprasylvian gyri—span regions in which areas of primarily visual (area 19) and somatic (area 5) provenance lie in contiguity with area 7. Area 7 is likely to be a region of convergence of auditory and somatic modalities since it receives fibres from area 5 and from the suprasylvian fringe. In the remaining polysensory area at the caudal end of the middle suprasylvian gyrus, area 19 is separated from area 7 only by the narrow unnamed area ("area 21") intercalated between the two and which, from the point of view of cortico-cortical connexions, is a part of the cortical visual system. In the two polysensory areas which have been extensively studied with micro-electrodes (the anterior middle suprasylvian and the anterior lateral areas), some neurons are modality specific for somatic, auditory or visual stimuli and many of the latter depend upon a cortico-cortical input from the visual cortex. Others are independent of the primary sensory cortex (Buser and Imbert, 1961; Dubner, 1966; Dubner and Rutledge, 1965; Buser and Imbert, 1961; Rutledge and Shellenberger, 1968). Therefore, we should like to suggest, tentatively, that the polymodal cells in these areas could belong to area 7 and that the uni-modal cells could lie in the contiguous "modality specific" fields. Despite this, it is still not possible to determine the exact route taken by impulses in reaching the polysensory areas since they are said to survive bilateral ablation of virtually all the cortex except the middle suprasylvian gyrus of one side (Thompson, Johnson and Hoopes, 1963) but to be independent of most of the thalamus as well (Bignall, Imbert and Buser, 1966; Bignall, 1967). They are, thus, independent of the only known thalamic input to area 7. One wonders, however, whether the overlap of cortico-thalamic projections from areas 5 and 7 and the four visual areas in the lateralis posterior nucleus may not be in some manner involved. This is particularly so as fibres from the superior colliculus end in the lateralis posterior nucleus and those visually activated cells in the anterior middle suprasylvian polysensory area which are independent of the visual cortex, show response properties similar to those in the superior colliculus (Dow and Dubner, 1969).

The coincidence of the polysensory areas and the areas of maximum barbiturate spindling and recruiting responses (Thompson, 1967) also has no obvious anatomical basis but a few points of possible relevance may be mentioned. The spindling effect and recruiting response are related to the midline and intralaminar thalamic nuclei and recruiting responses may also be obtained by stimulation of the posterior group "in the vicinity of the nucleus suprageniculatus" (Jasper, 1960). Area 7 is related by cortico-thalamic fibres to parts of both the intralaminar system (the central lateral nucleus) and the posterior group (the nucleus limitans and the suprageniculate nucleus); the suprageniculate nucleus and probably adjacent parts of the posterior group project to the suprasylvian fringe (Heath and Jones, 1971a) which, in turn, sends fibres to area 7. Finally, Thompson (1962) observed that the thalamic distribution of "association" responses of the type found in the polysensory areas, encompassed the *centre médian*, midline and ventro-anterior nuclei and the rostral midbrain reticular formation. There is, clearly, a relationship between all these parts of the thalamus and cortex but the actual mechanism of production of barbiturate spindling and of recruiting responses remains obscure.

The significance of interhemispheric fibres in sensory convergence has not yet been considered. From the present results and from many other studies of the commissural connexions of the neocortex, it would appear that there are few opportunities for multisensory convergence to occur by this route. Callosal fibres seem to provide for interhemispheric convergence *within* a sensory system: for example, SI projects to the opposite SI and SII (Jones and Powell, 1968c, 1969c), AI to the opposite AI and AII (Diamond et al., 1969) and areas 17, 18 and 19 all send fibres to the opposite lateral suprasylvian area as well as to their counterparts (Hubel and Wiesel, 1965; Garey et al., 1968; Wilson, 1968). (This should be qualified by the fact that certain important parts of the representation, such as that of the distal aspects of the limbs or of the periphery of the visual field, are not commissurally connected.) There are, however, no interhemispheric fibres *between* cortical areas related primarily to one sensory system and those related to another. Outside the primary sensory areas, the remaining areas of the cortex appear to be either connected solely to their counterparts or not commissurally connected at all. The lack of commissural connexions exhibited by the greater part of area 7 and by the insular and temporal cortex (Ebner and Myers, 1965; Diamond et al., 1969; present study) is particularly striking but at the moment, the significance of this lack of commissural connexions is quite obscure.

Output to the Limbic System

There are several main routes whereby activity emanating from the suprasylvian gyrus may enter the limbic system. One of the heaviest projections is from area 7 to the cingulate cortex, and this confirms Cragg's (1965) observations.

Since the somatic and auditory pathways appear to converge in area 7, this is an obvious route whereby such information may reach the hippocampus and, ultimately, the hypothalamus. Another pathway whereby different types of sensory information may reach the hippocampus is *via* the projections of areas 7, 20, Ep, the temporal area and the area intercalated between areas 7 and 19 to the peri-rhinal cortex (area 35). A less direct pathway would be from the various areas of the suprasylvian gyrus to the frontal lobe and back to the cingulate and retrosplenial areas (Cat 69). Finally, there is the projection from area 20 to the basolateral amygdala and it is interesting to note that close inter-relationship between the pulvinar, area 20 and the amygdala: the pulvinar projects to area 20 and to the basolateral amygdala (see also Graybiel, 1970) and area 20 sends fibres to both the pulvinar and the same part of the amygdala. All of the connexions of the suprasylvian gyrus and related areas with the limbic system, have their counterparts in the monkey (Jones and Powell, 1970a) and their possible function in sending "modality specific" and convergent sensory information to the hippocampus has been discussed elsewhere (Jones and Powell, 1970a). The important point to be noted here, is that the situations in the suprasylvian gyrus of the cat and in the parieto-temporal region of the monkey are identical.

Comparison with the Monkey

The pattern of cortico-cortical connexions of the suprasylvian gyrus closely resembles that in the parieto-temporal region of the rhesus monkey (Jones, 1969; Jones and Powell, 1970a). In the monkey, each primary sensory area has a projection to a local parieto-temporal field (which receives fibres from that sensory area alone) and a projection to a specific field of the frontal cortex. The frontal and local fields are then reciprocally connected. These steps are repeated until, ultimately, the three intracortical pathways emanating from the somatic, visual and auditory sensory cortices, converge in the depths of the superior temporal sulcus and in the orbito-frontal cortex of the frontal lobe. The auditory and visual paths also meet at the tip of the temporal lobe and this, and the orbito-frontal cortex, are interconnected. As the pathways converge, they commence sending fibres into parts of the limbic cortex, both in the cingulate gyrus and in the peri-rhinal area. Area 20 also sends fibres to the amygdala. The situation in the cat, although in some respects simpler, has obvious similarities with this pattern. The main points of difference are: there is far less differentiation of fields in the frontal lobe, so that many of the projections from the suprasylvian gyrus to area 6 overlap and apparently converge at a much earlier stage in the stepwise progression than in the monkey; the reciprocal connexion of each of the equivalent steps in the cortico-cortical progression in the parieto-temporal and frontal lobes are not so apparent in the cat, where fewer fibres seem to be returned to the suprasylvian regions from the frontal lobe; although a region of convergence between the cortico-cortical outputs of the visual and auditory systems is present in the cat, extending from the fundus of the posterior suprasylvian sulcus to the rhinal sulcus, this does not become continuous with the overlap and equivalent step in the progression from the somatic sensory cortex, as in the superior temporal sulcus of the monkey. Despite these differences, the number of steps proceeding outwards from the primary sensory areas is the same in the suprasylvian region of the cat as it is in the parieto-temporal region of the monkey and projections are sent to the cingulate and peri-rhinal areas and to the amygdala at the same points.

At first sight, area 7 presents another problem in the cat because projections of area 5 and the suprasylvian fringe seem to converge in it. In the monkey, Jones and Powell (1970a) found that area 5 sent fibres to area 7 but that the latter received no fibres from other fields. However, the discrepancy is probably due to the fact that the equivalent of the suprasylvian fringe was not damaged in any of the experiments in monkeys. After lesions involving the upper part of the superior temporal gyrus (area 22), Pandya and Kuypers (1969) observed axonal degeneration in area 7. In the experiments of Jones and Powell (1970a), lesions of area 22 were restricted to the lower part of the gyrus and no degeneration appeared in area 7. From this, we would suggest that the equivalent of the suprasylvian fringe in the monkey lies in the upper part of the superior temporal gyrus and possibly in the adjacent lateral and superior temporal sulci. The projections of area 5 and the suprasylvian fringe would overlap in area 7 of both the cat and monkey but whether they are actually congruent is difficult to determine. If they are not, this might account for the Vogt's (1919) and Bonin and Bailey's (1947) differentiation of area 7 in the monkey into rostral and caudal subareas (areas 7b or PF and 7a or PG respectively), and for Sanides and Hoffmann's (1969) subdivision of the approximately equivalent area in the cat into subareas Itsa and Itsp.

We consider that it is possible on the basis of similarities in connexions, to draw a close parallel between the suprasylvian gyrus of the cat and the parieto-temporal region of the monkey and to identify homologous fields, although in doing so, we are aware that, phylogenetically, a brain of the carnivore type was almost certainly never antecedent to that of the primate.

From the similarities in their patterns of connexions, it appears that the suprasylvian gyrus of the cat is the equivalent of the parieto-temporal region of the primate and that, in it, are situated many of the same cortical fields as are found in the higher primates. Probably, in their attempts to relate the cortical areas of all mammals to the multiple cortical "organs" which they felt they were demonstrating in man, early students of architectonics may have seen some homologous fields where none really existed. However, certain fields show remarkable constancy by being present and having the same relative dispositions in a wide range of mammals, even when delineated by workers who were not of the Vogt-Brodmann school. Among these, in addition to the main sensory areas, are particularly areas 5, 7, 20, 21 and 22 which have been described even in primitive insectivores. It seems significant that these are just the areas which stand in closest relationship to the primary sensory areas and which form the first and second steps in an outward cortico-cortical progression from the sensory areas (Jones and Powell, 1970a; present study). Hence, phylogenetic expansion may consist of the successive addition of new steps to the sequence.

On ascending the phylogenetic scale to man, in concert with the progressive enlargement of the neocortex, there is a small increase in the number of fields which have been described in the parieto-temporal region (Brodmann, 1909; Von Economo and Koskinas, 1925). However, as far as they have been studied, the cortico-cortical connexions of the association cortex of the cat and monkey are, up to a point, identical. The question, therefore, arises as to whether the same number of cortico-cortical connexions as in man are actually present in subhuman species, for, if so, the same number of fields could be present although unrecognized in being smaller. Therefore, the functional superiority of the human brain as reflected in the size of the cortex, could reflect an enlargement of already extant fields and of local connexions within them, rather than the addition of new fields and further steps in the chain of cortico-cortical connexions. Hence, in the buried cortex of the superior temporal sulcus of the monkey or of the posterior suprasylvian sulcus of the cat, several fields and cortico-cortical links could lie hidden. Alternatively, the areas in the depths of these sulci may be areas of ultimate convergence out of which new fields and, therefore, new cortico-cortical steps crystallize in phylogeny. It is assumed, however, that any new step will also acquire specific thalamic connexions and will not stand isolated from ascending sensory and other activity as was once thought for the "association cortex" (see Diamond and Hall, 1969).

Summary

The thalamic, associational and commissural connexions of the suprasylvian gyrus of the cat have been studied by means of the Nauta technique. Individual cortical fields were identified on the basis of their connexions and were correlated with existing functional and architectonic subdivisions of the gyrus. The parcellation of the gyrus on the basis of connexions (Fig. 22) agrees quite closely in those parts in which existing architectonic maps are in agreement with one another but diverges quite considerably in those parts in which the architectonic maps are in disagreement. The latter is particularly noticeable in regions in which there are no clear-cut architectonic boundaries.

The relationships of the fields in the suprasylvian gyrus to the primary sensory areas and to the thalamic sensory relay nuclei, were examined and the pattern of connexions was found to resemble quite closely that of the association cortex in the parieto-temporal region of the monkey.

The dorsal lateral geniculate nucleus projects directly to areas 17 and 18 of the visual cortex and these areas are reciprocally connected in an organized fashion with area 19 on the medial, and the lateral suprasylvian area on the lateral aspect of the suprasylvian gyrus. The major, and probably the sole thalamic input to area 19 and the lateral suprasylvian area is from the lateral nuclear complex of the thalamus. Area 19 and the lateral suprasylvian area are also reciprocally connected and area 19 sends fibres to an area ("area 20") at the inferior end of the posterior suprasylvian gyrus. Area 20 projects in turn to the amygdala, to the peri-rhinal cortex and to an area ("area 21") at the junction of the middle and posterior suprasylvian gyri. Both areas 20 and 21 are connected with the pulvinar of the thalamus. Area 21 and the lateral suprasylvian area send fibres to an area in the fundus of the posterior suprasylvian sulcus, to which area Ep of the auditory cortex also projects. This appears to be the homologue of a similar area of convergence in the depths of the superior temporal sulcus of the monkey.

The medial geniculate body projects directly to areas AI, AII, Ep and temporal of the auditory cortex and the first three of these send fibres to the suprasylvian fringe. (The suprasylvian fringe, with the insula, is the cortical target of certain parts of the posterior group of thalamic nuclei.) The suprasylvian fringe then projects to area 7 of the middle suprasylvian and lateral gyri.

The ventroposterior nucleus projects directly to areas SI and SII of the somatic sensory cortex and SI sends fibres to area 5 at the rostral ends of the middle suprasylvian and lateral gyri. Area 5, in turn, sends fibres to area 7, the projection overlapping with that of the suprasylvian fringe. The main efferent connexions of area 7 are with the cingulate cortex, the peri-rhinal cortex and the frontal lobe.

Most of the cortical areas in the suprasylvian gyrus have efferent connexions with area 6 of the frontal lobe and there is considerable overlap of these connexions in area 6. In some cases, reciprocal connexions are effected by fibres returning from the frontal lobe.

With the exception of area 7 which has few or no commissural connexions, all areas of the suprasylvian gyrus are commissurally connected with their homotopical areas in the opposite hemisphere. The lateral suprasylvian area receives callosal fibres from all four visual areas of the opposite side but sends fibres only to its counterpart.

None of the cortical areas defined on the basis of connexions in the suprasylvian gyrus, could be equated with the "polysensory areas". In these areas, in cats anaesthetized with chloralose, convergence upon single neurons of somatic, auditory and visual impulses, has been demonstrated. But cortico-cortical pathways related to the three sensory systems do not converge in or near the polysensory areas of the suprasylvian or lateral gyri. However, each of these polysensory areas is situated where narrow areas related to each of the three sensory systems lie in close contiguity. There is the possibility of convergence in the suprasylvian gyrus being mediated by the lateral nuclear-pulvinar complex since all sensory systems terminate in the superior colliculus and this is the main source of afferents to the lateral nuclear-pulvinar complex. A possible indication of such convergence is the marked overlap in the n. lateralis posterior exhibited by cortico-thalamic connexions emanating from many of the suprasylvian areas and from the visual cortex.

Acknowledgements. This work was supported by a grant from the New Zealand Medical Research Council. We are indebted to Dr. A. J. Rockel for assistance with some of the experiments and to Patricia Davey and Margaret Ogilvie for technical and artistic assistance.

References

Altman, J., Carpenter, M. B.: Fiber projections of the superior colliculus in the cat. J. comp. Neurol. 116, 157–177 (1961).
— Some fiber connections to the superior colliculus in the cat. J. comp. Neurol. 119, 77–96 (1962).
Bailey, P., Bonin, G. von: The isocortex of man. Urbana, Ill.: University of Illinois Press 1951.
Berlucchi, G., Gazzaniga, M. S., Rizzolati, G.: Microelectrode analysis of transfer of visual information by the corpus callosum. Arch. ital. Biol. 105, 583–598 (1967).
Bignall, K. E.: Comparison of optic afferents to primary visual and polysensory areas of cat neocortex. Exp. Neurol. 17, 327–343 (1967).
— Imbert, M.: Polysensory and cortico-cortical projections to frontal lobe of squirrel and rhesus monkey. Electroenceph. clin. Neurophysiol. 26, 206–215 (1969).
— — Buser, P.: Optic projections to nonvisual cortex of the cat. J. Neurophysiol. 29, 396–409 (1966).

Bishop, G. H.: The relation between nerve fiber size and sensory modality: phylogenetic implications of the afferent innervation of cortex. J. nerv. ment. Dis. 128, 89–114 (1959).

Blomquist, A. J., Lorenzini, C. A.: Projection of dorsal roots and sensory nerves to cortical sensory motor regions of squirrel monkey. J. Neurophysiol. 28, 1195–1205 (1965).

Bonin, G. von., Bailey, P.: The neocortex of Macaca Mulatta. Urbana, Ill.: University of Illinois Press 1947.

Brodmann, K.: Vergleichende Lokalisationslehre der Großhirnrinde in ihren Prinzipien dargestellt auf Grund des Zellenbaues, 1st ed. Leipzig: J. A. Barth 1909.

Burrows, G. R., Hayhow, W. R.: Thalamo-cortical relationships in cat visual system. J. Anat. (Lond.) 106, 205–206 (1970).

Burton, H., Earls, F.: Cortical representation of the ipsilateral chorda tympani nerve in the cat. Brain Res. 16, 520–523 (1969).

Buser, P., Bignall, K. E.: Nonprimary sensory projections on cat neocortex. Int. Rev. Neurobiol. 10, 111–165 (1967).

Choudhury, B. P., Whitteridge, D., Wilson, M. E.: The function of the callosal connections of the visual cortex. Quart. J. exp. Physiol. 50, 214–219 (1965).

Clare, M. H., Bishop, G. H.: Responses from an association area secondarily activated from optic cortex. J. Neurophysiol. 17, 271–277 (1954).

Clark, W. E. Le Gros: A note on cortical cyto-architectonics. Brain 75, 96–104 (1952).

— Powell, T. P. S.: On the thalamo-cortical connexions of the general sensory cortex of Macaca. Proc. roy. Soc. B 141, 467–487.

Clüver, P. F. de V., Campos-Ortega, J. A.: The cortical projection of the pulvinar in the cat. J. comp. Neurol. 137, 295–307 (1969).

Cragg, B. G.: Afferent connexions of the allocortex. J. Anat. (Lond.) 99, 339–357 (1965).

Darian-Smith, I., Isbister, J., Mok, H., Yokota, T.: Somatic sensory cortical projection areas excited by tactile stimulation of the cat: a triple representation. J. Physiol. (Lond.) 182, 671–689 (1966).

Diamond, I. T., Hall, W. C.: Evolution of neocortex. Science 164, 251–262 (1969).

— Jones, E. G., Powell, T. P. S.: The association connections of the auditory cortex of the cat. Brain Res. 11, 560–579 (1968a).

— — — Interhemispheric fiber connections of the auditory cortex of the cat. Brain Res. 11, 177–193 (1968b).

— — — The projection of the auditory cortex upon the diencephalon and brain stem in the cat. Brain Res. 15, 305–340 (1969).

Dow, B. M., Dubner, R.: Visual receptive fields and responses to movement in an association area of cat cerebral cortex. J. Neurophysiol. 32, 773–784 (1969).

Dubner, R.: Single cell analysis of sensory interaction in anterior lateral and suprasylvian gyri of the cat cerebral cortex. Exp. Neurol. 15, 255–273 (1966).

— Brown, F. J.: Response of cells to restricted visual stimuli in an association area of cat cerebral cortex. Exp. Neurol. 20, 70–86 (1968).

— Rutledge, L. T.: Recording and analysis of converging input upon neurons in cat association cortex. J. Neurophysiol. 27, 620–634 (1964).

— — Intracellular recording of the convergence of input upon neurons in cat association cortex. Exp. Neurol. 12, 349–369 (1965).

Ebner, F. F., Myers, R. E.: Distribution of corpus callosum and anterior commissure in cat and raccoon. J. comp. Neurol. 124, 353–366 (1965).

Economo, C. von, Koskinas, G. N.: Die Cytoarchitektonik der Hirnrinde des erwachsenen Menschen. Vienna and Berlin: Springer 1925.

Fink, R. P., Heimer, L.: Two methods for selective silver impregnation of degenerating axons and their synaptic endings in the central nervous system. Brain Res. 4, 369–374 (1967).

Garey, L. J., Jones, E. G., Powell, T. P. S.: Interrelationships of striate and extrastriate cortex with the primary relay sites of the visual pathway. J. Neurol. Neurosurg. Psychiat. 31, 135–157 (1968).

— Powell, T. P. S.: The projection of the lateral geniculate nucleus upon the cortex in the cat. Proc. roy. Soc. B 169, 107–126 (1967).

Glickstein, M., King, R. A., Miller, J., Berkley, M.: Cortical projections from the dorsal lateral geniculate nucleus of cats. J. comp. Neurol. 130, 55–76 (1967).

Graybiel, A. M.: Some thalamocortical projections of the pulvinar-posterior system of the thalamus in the cat. Brain Res. **22**, 131–136 (1970).

Guillery, R. W.: Patterns of fiber degeneration in the dorsal lateral geniculate nucleus of the cat following lesions in the visual cortex. J. comp. Neurol. **130**, 197–222 (1967).

Gurewitsch, M., Chatschaturian, A.: Zur Cytoarchitektonik der Großhirnrinde der Feliden. Z. Anat. Entwickl.-Gesch. **87**, 100–138 (1928).

Hassler, R., Muhs-Clement, K.: Architektonischer Aufbau des sensomotorischen und parietalen Cortex der Katze. J. Hirnforsch. **6**, 377–420 (1964).

Heath, C. J.: Distribution of axonal degeneration following lesions of the posterior group of thalamic nuclei in the cat. Brain Res. **21**, 435–438 (1970).

— Jones, E. G.: Connexions of area 19 and the lateral suprasylvian area of the visual cortex of the cat. Brain Res. **19**, 302–305 (1970).

— — An experimental study of ascending connections from the posterior group of thalamic nuclei in the cat. J. comp. Neurol. **141**, 397–426 (1971).

Holländer, H.: The projection from the visual cortex to the lateral geniculate body (LGB). An experimental study with silver impregnation methods in the cat. Exp. Brain Res. **10**, 219–235 (1970).

Hubel, D. H., Wiesel, T. N.: Receptive fields and functional architecture in two non-striate visual areas (18 and 19) of the cat. J. Neurophysiol. **28**, 229–289 (1965).

— — Cortical and callosal connections concerned with the vertical meridian of visual fields in the cat. J. Neurophysiol. **30**, 1561–1573 (1967).

— — Visual area of the lateral suprasylvian gyrus (Clare-Bishop area) of the cat. J. Physiol. (Lond.) **202**, 251–260 (1969).

Jasper, H. H.: Unspecific thalamocortical relations. In: Handbook of physiology, sect. 1, Neurophysiology, vol. 2, p. 1307–1321. Washington DC: American Physiological Soc. 1960.

Jassik-Gerschenfeld, D.: Activity of somatic origin evoked in the superior colliculus of the cat. Exp. Neurol. **16**, 104–118 (1966).

Jones, E. G.: Interrelationships of parieto-temporal and frontal cortex in the rhesus monkey Brain Res. **13**, 412–415 (1969).

— Powell, T. P. S.: The ipsilateral cortical connexions of the somatic sensory areas in the cat. Brain Res. **9**, 71–94 (1968a).

— — The projection of the somatic sensory cortex upon the thalamus in the cat. Brain Res. **10**, 369–391 (1968b).

— — The commissural connexions of the somatic sensory cortex in the cat. J. Anat. (Lond.) **103**, 433–455 (1968c).

— — Connexions of the somatic sensory cortex of the rhesus monkey. I. Ipsilateral cortical connexions. Brain **92**, 477–502 (1969a).

— — The cortical projection of the ventroposterior nucleus of the thalamus in the cat. Brain Res. **13**, 298–318 (1969b).

— — Connexions of the somatic sensory cortex of the rhesus monkey. II. Contralateral cortical connexions. Brain **92**, 717–730 (1969c).

— — An experimental study of converging sensory pathways in the cerebral cortex of the monkey. Brain **93**, 793–820 (1970a).

— — Connexions of the somatic sensory cortex of the rhesus monkey. III. Thalamic connexions. Brain **93**, 37–56 (1970b).

— — An analysis of the posterior group of thalamic nuclei on the basis of its afferent connections. J. comp. Neurol. (in press) (1971).

Kaas, J., Hall, W. C., Diamond, I. T.: Cortical visual areas I and II in the hedgehog: relation between evoked potential maps and architectonic subdivisions. J. Neurophysiol. **33**, 59–5615 (1970).

Kuypers, H. G. J., M., Lawrence, D. G.: Cortical projections to the red nucleus and the brain stem in the rhesus monkey. Brain Res. **4**, 151–188 (1967).

Landgren, S., Silfvenius, H.: Projections of the eye and the neck region on the anterior suprasylvian cerebral cortex of the cat. Acta physiol. scand. **74**, 340–347 (1968).

— — Wolsk, D.: Vestibular, cochlear and trigeminal projections to the cortex in the anterior suprasylvian sulcus of the cat. J. Physiol. (Lond.) **191**, 561–573 (1967).

Lashley, K. S., Clark, G.: The cytoarchitecture of the cerebral cortex of *Ateles:* a critical examination of architectonic studies. J. comp. Neurol. **85**, 223–305 (1946).

Mehler, W. R.: Some neurological species differences — *a posteriori*. Ann. N. Y. Acad. Sci. **167**, 424–468 (1969).

Mickle, W. A., Ades, H. W.: A composite sensory projection area in the cerebral cortex of the cat. Amer. J. Physiol. **170**, 682–689 (1952).

Nauta, W. J. H., Gygax, P. A.: Silver impregnation of degenerating axons in the central nervous system: a modified technic. Stain Technol. **29**, 91–93 (1954).

— Kuypers, H. G. J. M.: Some ascending pathways in the brain stem reticular foundation. In: Reticular formation of the brain, p. 3–30, eds. H. H. Jasper, L. D. Proctor, R. S. Knighton, W. C. Noshay and R. T. Costello. Boston: Little, Brown & Co 1958.

Niimi, K., Sprague, J. M.: Thalamo-cortical organization of the visual system in the cat. J. comp. Neurol. **138**, 219–249 (1970).

Otsuka, R., Hassler, R.: Über Aufbau und Gliederung der corticalen Sehsphäre bei der Katze. Arch. Psychiat. Nervenkr. **203**, 212–234 (1962).

Pandya, D., Kuypers, H. G. J. M.: Cortico-cortical connections in the rhesus monkey. Brain Res. **13**, 13–36 (1969).

Penfield, W., Jasper, H.: Epilepsy and the functional anatomy of the human brain. Boston: Little, Brown & Co. 1954.

Powell, T. P. S., Mountcastle, V. B.: Some aspects of the functional organization of the cortex of the postcentral gyrus of the monkey: a correlation of findings obtained in a single unit analysis with cytoarchitecture. Bull. Johns Hopk. Hosp. **105**, 133–162 (1959).

Rioch, D. McK.: Studies on the diencephalon of carnivora. Part I. The nuclear configuration of the thalamus, epthalamus and hypothalamus of the dog and cat. J. comp. Neurol. **49**, 1–119 (1929).

Roberts, T. S., Akert, K.: Insular and opercular cortex and its thalamic projection in *Macaca Mulatta*. Schweiz. Arch. Neurol. Neurochir. Psychiat. **92**, 1–43 (1963).

Rose, J. E., Woolsey, C. N.: The orbitofrontal cortex and its connections with the mediodorsal nucleus in rabbit, sheep and cat. Res. Publ. Ass. nerv. ment. Dis. **27**, 210–232 (1948a).

— — Structure and relations of limbic cortex and anterior thalamic nuclei in rabbit and cat. J. comp. Neurol. **89**, 279–347 (1948b).

— — Organization of the mammalian thalamus and its relationships to the cerebral cortex. Electroenceph. clin. Neurophysiol. **1**, 391–403 (1949a).

— — The relations of thalamic connections, cellular structure and evocable electrical activity in the auditory region of the cat. J. comp. Neurol. **91**, 441–466 (1949b).

— — Cortical connections and functional organization of the thalamic auditory system in the cat. In: Biological and biochemical bases of behavior, p. 127–150, eds. H. F. Harlow and C. N. Woolsey. Madison, Wis.: University of Wisconsin Press 1958.

Rutledge, L. T., Shellenberger, M. K.: The influence of visual cortex upon nonprimary area neurons. Arch. ital. Biol. **106**, 353–363 (1968).

Sanides, F., Hoffmann, J.: Cyto- and myeloarchitecture of the visual cortex of the cat and of the surrounding integration cortices. J. Hirnforsch. **11**, 79–104 (1969).

— Krishnamurti, A.: Cytoarchitectonic subdivisions of sensorimotor and prefrontal regions and of bordering insular and limbic fields in slow loris (*Nycticebus coucang coucang*). J. Hirnforsch. **9**, 226–252 (1967).

Schneider, G. E.: Two visual systems. Science **163**, 891–895 (1969).

Thompson, R. F.: Thalamocortical organisation of association responses to auditory, tactile and visual stimuli in cat. Intern. Congr. Physiol. Sci. 21st Series No 48, p. 1057. Leiden 1962.

— Foundations of physiological psychology, p. 474–528. New York-Evanston-London: Harper and Row 1967.

— Johnson, R. H., Hoopes, J. J.: Organization of auditory, somatic sensory and visual projection to association fields of cerebral cortex in the cat. J. Neurophysiol. **26**, 343–364 (1963).

Vogt, C., Vogt, O.: Allgemeinere Ergebnisse unserer Hirnforschung. J. Psychol. Neurol. **25**. 277–462 (1919).

Waller, W. H., Barris, R. W.: Relationships of thalamic nuclei to the cerebral cortex in the cat. J. comp. Neurol. 67, 317–341 (1937).

Walzl, E. M., Mountcastle, V. B.: Projection of vestibular nerve to cerebral cortex of cat. Amer. J. Physiol. 159, 595 (1949).

Weiskrantz, L.: Experiments on the r.n.s. (real nervous system) and monkey memory. Proc. roy. Soc. B 171, 335–352 (1968).

Wilson, M. E.: Cortico-cortical connexions of the cat visual areas. J. Anat. (Lond.) 102, 375–386 (1968).

— Cragg, B. G.: Projections from the lateral geniculate nucleus in the cat and monkey. J. Anat. (Lond.) 101, 677–692 (1967).

Woollard, H. H., Harpman, J. A.: The connexions of the inferior colliculus and of the dorsal nucleus of the lateral lemniscus. J. Anat. (Lond.) 74, 441–458 (1940).

Woolsey, C. N.: The somatic functions of the central nervous system. Ann. Rev. Physiol. 9, 525–552 (1947).

— Organization of somatic sensory and motor areas of the cerebral cortex. In: Biological and biochemical bases of behavior, p. 63–81, eds. H. F. Harlow and C. N. Woolsey. Madison, Wis.: University of Wisconsin Press 1958.

— Organization of cortical auditory system. In: Principles of sensory communication, p. 235–257, ed. W. A. Rosenblith. Cambridge, Mass.: M.I.T. Press 1961.

Wright, M. J.: Visual receptive fields of cells in a cortical area remote from the striate cortex in the cat. Nature (Lond.) 223, 973–975 (1969).

Subject Index